3X WEIGHT LOSS

HOW TO LOSE WEIGHT 3X FASTER AND KEEP IT OFF FOR GOOD WITHOUT STARVING, CRAVINGS, OR WILLPOWER!

By

Laura Sales

DEDICATION

To my husband, Tim, who opened my eyes to a whole new world of health and wellness and who led the way to the discoveries found in this book. Thank you for the relentless love, encouragement and support that you have given me in realizing my dreams. You are my rock. My hero. My everything. Without you none of this would have been made possible.

And to our boys, Braxton and Tristan, you two are my greatest accomplishments and it is such an honor to be your mama. I couldn't have been more blessed to have you in my life. Thank you for being you and for choosing me.

FOREWORD

By Dr. Ray Strand

I have been involved in a private family practice for over 40 years. One of the most difficult and frustrating problems I have had to deal with over the years is trying to help my patients, especially women, who desire to lose weight. Researching the medical literature in hopes of finding an answer only led to more frustration as I realized that even if my patients were able to lose weight with one of the popular diets, 98% of them would gain that weight back and usually more within two years.

So the question I began asking myself was: Why do diets fail so often? Well, the main reason diets fail is the fact that they are a short-term solution for a long-term problem. The connotation when any of my patients would tell me that they are going to be going on such-and-such diet was the fact that somewhere in the future they would be coming off that diet and usually returning to those poor lifestyles that got them into this problem in the beginning. Another major reason that diets fail is because they are not healthy. They eliminate all the carbohydrates or all the fats in an attempt to help people lose weight. The problem is that they can't stay on these diets long term because they are NOT healthy. So what is the answer to this dilemma? Well, it is not going to be another diet that the medical literature has shown me will fail 98% of the time. This would simply be a waste of our time.

My patients had to learn that the most important drug they take into their body is the foods they choose to eat. Eating the wrong foods sets off a hormonal response that leads to uncontrollable hunger, increased inflammation in their bodies, and over time tips them over into an abnormal metabolic state. When my patients finally tipped over into this abnormal metabolic state, they were unable to utilize the calories they ate effectively. Instead of using their calories from their food as energy, the body was now storing most of those calories as fat. They actually held on to this fat like a sponge holds on to water. In fact, if my patients were not able to firmly establish healthy lifestyles to bring their bodies back into balance, they were not able to lose weight effectively and permanently. However, the primary concern for my patients was not the fact that they were not able to lose weight, but that this abnormal metabolic state was also causing them to lose their health.

3X Weight Loss is a scientifically based program. It only makes common sense that if it has been our poor lifestyles that have gotten us into this situation, then firmly establishing healthy lifestyles can get us out of this situation. This is the essence of the 3X Weight Loss Program. It is NOT another diet. 3X guides you into firmly establishing new, healthier lifestyles that bring your body back into balance and allows you to begin releasing excessive fat effectively.

As a physician, I am excited about the 3X Weight Loss Program because as you begin releasing fat you will also begin to see your health improve. Participants have noted improvement in their blood pressure, blood sugar, cholesterol levels, inflammation, sleep patterns, energy, and focus.

Participants of the 3X Program have shared with me that they feel they have found something they can finally stick to and get results. They say things like, "What is so hard about never going hungry, feeling great, having more energy and focus, seeing your health parameters improve, and oh yes, beginning to lose excessive fat when you are not really trying?" Why are you not trying? Because the 3X Weight Loss Program does not rely on willpower. 3X guides you into firmly establishing those healthy lifestyles that bring your body back into balance and allows you to tip back into a normal metabolic state. In other words, you will be correcting the underlying problem that got you into trouble in the first place. Since you are establishing new, healthier lifestyles and not going on another diet, you will continue what you learn in the 3X Weight Loss Program for the rest of your life. This is the reason 3X is different. No matter what your frustration has been in the past in regards to trying to lose weight, the 3X Weight Loss Program will give you the absolute best chance of establishing your healthy weight as you improve your health.

Dr. Ray Strand, MD
Author of "What Your Doctor Doesn't Know about Nutritional Medicine May be Killing You"

WHAT IS 3X WEIGHT LOSS?

Hi! I'm Laura Sales, a mother of two, a Certified Fitness Nutrition Specialist, and the creator of the 3X Weight Loss Program. Before we jump into the specifics of 3X Weight Loss, I'm going to tell you about my background, give insight into what the program is, and more importantly, what it is not.

The internet is loaded with free information about how to lose weight. Type in "How to lose weight" into Google and you will see a staggering 37,000,000 results pop up! And it doesn't stop with search results. Facebook, YouTube, and other social media sites are flooded with videos and ads from the latest diet guru or exercise enthusiast. Your local bookstore has thousands of books on weight loss. There is absolutely no shortage of information out there about how to lose weight and the last thing the world needs is another diet book filled with short-term diet advice, recipes, tips, and tricks!

You're probably thinking to yourself, "How is this book going to be any different, Laura?" Anyone can go on a diet, lose a few pounds, and get short-term results, but I'm not interested in teaching you how to do that. I want you to have the power to be in full control of your weight, be the master of your body, and to be free from dieting forever. And yes, those are achievable goals!

This is not the typical diet book that is going to simply provide you with a few recipes and send you on your way. This is a handbook that will guide, educate, and empower you with the knowledge you need to not only get the body you want, but make it so that you **never have to diet again**.

The reason that this program is called "3X Weight Loss" is because properly followed, you can realize results three times faster with this than on other diet and exercise programs.

Now, let me clarify what 3X Weight loss is not. 3X Weight Loss is **NOT** a quick fix to lose weight, yet the strategy I am going to share with you will help you lose exponentially more weight faster than ever before. 3X Weight Loss is NOT another short-term diet program, but a realistic lifestyle plan that you can maintain even after you've lost all your weight.

3X Weight Loss is **NOT** about exercising yourself to death to burn more calories than you consume, yet this book WILL help you burn deep into your fat stores without having to spend a minute in the gym. And last but not least, 3X Weight Loss is **NOT** about searching to find motivation, yet by the time you have finished reading this book, you will have more ambition to get healthy & lose weight than you've ever thought was possible.

I recently had the pleasure to work with a woman named Carrie. When she first contacted me she confided, "Laura, I really want to try your program, but I've failed so many times at losing weight and nothing seems to work for me. How is your program going to be any different?"

To better understand Carrie's specific situation, I asked her what her biggest challenge with losing weight was. Here is her response:

"Losing weight, period. I have been at a plateau for years now. I exercise every day, weights, running, cardio of all sorts. I watch what I eat as far as portion sizes goes. I am 46

and I weigh 164 and I am 5'3," kind of a stocky build and I am so discouraged. I don't know if I am starting menopause or what is going on, but if I get off track at all I put weight on immediately. I have been working on myself for eight and a half years and I feel like I should be so much farther than I am. I want to be lean and healthy not somewhat chunky, which is the way I feel. I have tried almost every diet out there and I still get nothing."

I then asked Carrie about her exercise routine and to send me exactly what she eats daily. She replied:

"My exercise in a day consists of 15–30 minutes of stair stepper or walking incline on the treadmill, sunny days I run on the street for 30–60 minutes.

On top of that, I do weight lifting of all sorts for 30–45 minutes.

I eat breakfast that is either steel cut oats with a tsp of butter, tsp of brown sugar and ½ cup of blueberries. Snack is a yogurt, lunch is two to three tbsps of hummus, one cup of carrots, ½ cup of tuna with a few cherry tomatoes, green onions, a little olive oil and lemon juice. Snack one oz of sharp cheddar cheese with six Triscuit crackers.

Dinner is usually a cooked chicken breast and spring salad mix with feta cheese, sunflower seeds, cherry tomatoes, a couple of croutons, onions, etc. and dressing is olive oil based, about two to three tbsps.

My evening snack is an apple and peanut butter. I drink at least ½ to one gallon of water daily. I do not drink soda, sweet tea, or anything else of the sort. Always water..."

After processing all of this information, I knew exactly what the problem was and why she wasn't able to lose any weight, despite how healthy her diet was. I could see right off of the bat with all that she had been doing for roughly the past decade that she definitely didn't have a motivation or willpower problem. I told her, "You're in luck. I know exactly what's going on and how to fix it. The good news is that you do not have a "weight loss" problem. You have a diet and exercise problem."

Like most women, the reason Carrie wasn't able to lose any weight, despite her many efforts, was because she was attempting to fix the wrong problem: her weight. Weight is actually just a symptom of a deeper underlying issue.

Carrie was following all the conventional diet and exercise advice and, in her mind, was doing everything right. Yet she thought there was something wrong with her body because she couldn't get results.

Carrie is not alone with these struggles. Countless women are in this situation, feeling hopeless and frustrated at their body's lack of responsiveness.

Would you like to know what changes I told Carrie to make to her diet and exercise routine? Or how you turn a body that is constantly storing fat despite dieting and exercising, into a body that burns fat 24 hours a day while eating more and exercising less? THAT is what this book is about. Have I got your attention now?

This book will take you on a journey that will teach you not only how to lose weight 3X faster without starving, cravings, or willpower, but also how to get extremely healthy in the process.

During this journey, I will expose many of the weight loss myths about diets and exercise that are keeping you from seeing the results you desire and how it really has nothing to do with motivation or willpower.

Once you understand the foundational concepts behind 3X Weight Loss, we'll dive into the specifics of the plan and explore the details you will need to implement this program into your life.

By the end of this book, you will never again wonder what you need to do to lose weight. You will be empowered with a new set of healthy habits to set up your lifestyle in a way that will give you more results in less time, with less stress, and with more freedom to do the things you want with your life. As a result, you'll feel a new sense of enthusiasm and passion for taking your body and health to the next level from knowing exactly where to focus your energy to get the best results.

This isn't to say you will always be perfect or that you need to be. Life happens, and you will get thrown off track here and there—we all do. Yet at the end of this book you'll be able to say to yourself, "I finally know exactly how to be the healthiest version of me so that I can lose weight naturally and keep it off for good. I'm confident in my ability to live a healthy lifestyle consistently and am prepared to overcome any adversity that will come my way!"

When you implement the strategies of this book, you will have set of powerful habits that reliably lead to optimal health and long-term weight loss success without you even having to think about it.

You reading this book makes it clear that you're serious about making a change. Hopefully, that is coupled with full dedication and commitment to implementing these strategies because you're about to enter a transformational period of your life; you're about to become a revitalized you from the inside out.

Now that you have a clear understanding of what 3X Weight Loss is and is not, I'm going to share with you who I am and what inspired me to write this book.

TABLE OF CONTENTS

INTRODUCTION

Interestingly enough, it was never my goal to be a weight loss coach or to be an expert in health, nutrition, or weight loss. And I definitely never intended on writing a book on the topic. In fact, just a few years ago, I was perfectly happy being a corporate professional turned stay-at-home mom and helping my husband with his business on the side. But I had a life-changing experience that lead me to become insanely passionate about health and wellness. I believe I have an important message that can help millions of women who are unnecessarily suffering with losing weight by essentially starving, taking dangerous diet pills, or by doing extreme exercise programs, and it has become a passion of mine to share it.

When it comes to losing weight, women have been completely duped and led down so many wrong paths. Each failure causes us to become more and more desperate to lose weight, to the point that we will try almost any quick fix promise, magic pill, or diet fad that is offered to us.

With what I now know about weight loss and how the body really works, it kills me to see the ridiculous diet suggestions that the most popular diet and exercise programs make. We are most definitely being set up to fail!

I know what it's like to wish you had a different body than what you have and to stare at other women who are toned and fit and to silently wish you could look like them. I know what it's like to daydream and picture in your mind what you hope to look like on the next vacation or pool party after you've done the next 60-day challenge, weight-loss program, diet, or cleanse. I know what it's like to try on outfit after outfit and feel hopeless because nothing looks good. I know what it's like to go shopping for new clothes, only to end up wanting to just cry in the dressing room. (What's up with those dressing room lights, anyway? They are horrible!)

I know what it's like to catch a glimpse of yourself in the mirror and wonder what happened to the cute-shaped girl you used to be, and then to be in complete denial that it's really you that you're looking at. I know what it's like to feel guilty about eating the piece of dark chocolate or for having a slice of pizza at the party, then to tell yourself, "The diet starts Monday," or, "I'll just try harder at the gym tomorrow."

After having my first baby I was diagnosed with high cholesterol, a low thyroid, and several other hormonal imbalances and nutritional deficiencies. This was actually quite shocking to me because, at the time, I considered myself to be one of the healthiest people I knew. I ate healthily, took a ton of vitamins, and I exercised 3-5 times a week. Despite my healthy lifestyle and young age though, I was 25 pounds overweight, was overly stressed, and exhausted all the time.

In an attempt to fix my health and weight problems, I decided to do what seemingly all experts recommend—eat less and exercise more. I started going to the gym every morning to do cardio on the treadmill. I hired a personal trainer, attended fitness classes, and paid for expensive meal plan delivery services.

I did cleanses, shake diets, detoxes and even the body wraps!

No matter what I tried it seemed like my body had turned against me because I couldn't get the results I wanted and the things that worked for me in the past (before having kids) no longer did.

Every time I thought I was making progress I would start to get excited. But as soon as I ate anything even remotely off the diet, every pound that I lost came right back. It was a vicious cycle that made me feel like I was always taking one step forward and two steps backward. I just couldn't understand why all of a sudden, my body stopped working the way it used to.

Since these "tried and true" strategies of eating less and exercising more obviously weren't working for me, I began to do my own research into nutrition and weight loss for the first time. I just knew there had to be an approach that I hadn't tried and wasn't willing to accept being overweight and unhealthy for the rest of my life.

As a result, I became a Certified Fitness Nutrition Specialist and spent two years researching and studying the topics of nutrition and weight loss. I read over 40 diet books and I sifted through thousands of weight loss articles and read through hundreds of clinical studies. I even consulted personally with doctors, clinical nutritionists, naturopaths, homeopaths, supplement formulators, personal trainers, and more.

During my journey, I learned something that not a lot of people in the mainstream weight loss space are talking about. I learned that **fat is a symptom of a deeper underlying issue in the body**. Factually, there is scientific a reason why our bodies store fat in the first place, and it doesn't have to do with how many calories you're eating or how much exercise you're doing either. Of course, after following the mainstream advice of eating less and exercising more, 70% of the population is still overweight.

Here's what the dieting industry doesn't want you to know. You are already hardwired for a healthy, youthful, energetic body, and once you shift your attention to fixing the real cause instead of focusing on the symptom, your body will naturally rid itself of fat and weight will no longer be an issue for you.

It was such a sigh of relief when I finally discovered the real reason I couldn't lose weight. There was absolutely nothing wrong with me, I was simply trying to fix the wrong problem. I was focusing on losing fat, which was actually just a symptom of the real problem. Once I understood this, it made weight loss so much easier to understand.

Once I shifted my focus to fixing the cause instead of the symptom, I instantly saw results and my health improved practically overnight. My results were like night and day compared to my previous efforts. The weight literally fell off in a matter of weeks and I had more energy than I knew what to do with!

After I let go of my preconceived notions of what was "healthy," educated myself about basic nutrition and weight loss and discovered manageable eating and lifestyle strategies, I not only quit struggling to lose weight, but was finally able to consistently maintain a habit of health.

My story isn't the kind of transformation you'll see often see touted on the latest reality TV show or Weight Watchers advertisement. In my case, it took years to figure out not only how to reach my goals, but to maintain my "transformation." And while I lost 25 pounds of fat, gained muscle, and got my cholesterol and hormone levels back to normal, the real "before and after" is my mindset shift. Because in reality, the only weight-loss program that works is the one you stick with for life.

The most amazing part of my journey wasn't just about losing weight. The true benefit is knowing that I'm in control of my body. I know that moving forward, I will never have to diet again. I don't have to worry anymore about how to lose weight or wonder if I'm ever going to be able to fit back into my old clothes.

For example, a couple months ago, my husband and I went on a cruise and we ate like total crap for 10 days straight! We were eating the buffet food and a ton of desserts. And even between meals, we ate cookies and ice cream and all the bad stuff. What I knew in the back of my mind, though, was that the second I got home, I would be going back to my regular, healthy lifestyle. And that no matter how much weight I gained on the cruise, I would immediately lose it when I got home. That's control because I am able to still go out and enjoy my life. I can eat bad food if I want to, but I know exactly how I'm going to get back on track to get my body right back in balance.

This is what I want for you also. It is my goal that by the time you are finished reading this book, you too can start your journey to getting the permanent results you are looking for while still living your life and enjoying the entire process! Here we go!

SECTION 1

THE TRUTH ABOUT WEIGHT LOSS

CHAPTER 1

YOU CAN DO THIS

I f you're anything like the thousands of other women I've coached, you've definitely tried it all. The starvation diets, juice cleanses, shakes, and insane workout routines. Maybe you've even tried the body wraps, creams, potions, and lotions. You've been there, done that, and probably have a couple t-shirts to prove it!

Yet, regardless of all this, you still have a burning desire inside of you and a clear picture in your mind of exactly what you want to look like. And that vision is what keeps you searching for the answer. You know deep down that the truth is out there somewhere, you just have to find it. How do I know all of this? Because I've been there. I also know that you wouldn't be reading this book if you didn't think that it was somehow possible for you to achieve your goals.

If you are currently struggling to lose weight, you may *think* you have a motivation or willpower problem. You might even think there is something wrong with your body since losing weight has historically proven to be so difficult for you, but that is simply not the case. Your lack of results has nothing to do with willpower, motivation, counting calories, or exercise. After working with thousands of clients, I've found that low motivation, lack of willpower, and stubborn body fat are just symptoms of a much greater problem—one that's hard to see (the bad news), but a lot easier to fix (the good news).

No one is going to be able to stay on a program that isn't working and furthermore, there is no amount of motivation or willpower that can overcome the body's powerful built-in survival mechanisms for cravings and hunger. You see, when you go on a diet, your body immediately starts working against you. It doesn't know or care about weight loss; it only knows about survival, as that's its number one priority. Your body will not give up fat and will continue to make it as long as it thinks it is being threatened.

You can have all the ambition, motivation, and willpower in the world. You can try starvation diets and do rigorous exercise programs. You can have surgery, staple your stomach to make it smaller, or suck the fat out of your thighs with a vacuum. You can even inject yourself with hormones or take all sorts of drugs, stimulants, and synthetic vitamins. You can fight your body tooth and nail to lose weight, but it will *always* win. And as long as you are addressing the symptom, weight, this problem is guaranteed to come back no matter what you try.

I like to use the analogy of your car needing a repair. When the check engine light appears on the dashboard, most of us think, "Uh-oh. Something is wrong. I've got to make an appointment to take my car in for a repair." Sometimes, we even think that we can procrastinate a little bit and not call right away. We think that if there was something really wrong with the car, it wouldn't start, or we would see smoke coming out from under the hood. But nevertheless, the check engine light is our early warning sign that something needs our attention.

If we pop the hood, take out a pair of pliers, cut the wire to the check engine light and say, "This is fixed," do you think that that would really solve the issue with your car? Or do you think not handling the reason the light came on in the first place would cause it to get worse and even lead to other, more severe problems down the road?

Attempting to lose weight by counting calories, doing excessive exercise, taking appetite suppressants, getting surgery, or by taking injections is like cutting a wire to the check engine signal.

Having excess fat is a sign of deeper underlying issue in the body. Your body is storing fat for a reason, and you must address the root cause if you want to reach your ideal body weight and stay there. And let me make it very clear early on: Being overweight is not just a matter of fitting into your skinny jeans. It is not just a vanity issue. Fat is a symptom of a deeper, underlying issue within the body, and for every excess pound of fat that you have on your body, you are that much closer to what could be a life-threatening disease.

Here are some very important stats to consider:

- Women with a waist circumference over 35 inches are at increased risk of heart and other diseases.
- Women with a waist of 37 inches or more have an 80% higher risk of death than those with waists of 27 inches or less.
- Women with waists of 35 inches or higher have three times the risk of death from heart disease compared to normal women whose waists are smaller than 35 inches.

Not to mention being overweight can severely affect your quality of life. Again, this is not just about what you see when you look in the mirror.

THE BODY TIPPING POINT

This epidemic of having pesky, excess fat correlates to a concept I call "The Body Tipping Point," which I became aware of through coaching so many women to lose weight. It means that if you do not take this seriously, if you do not make your health a priority and get rid of this excess fat, it's only going to get worse. And it's only going to get harder.

When I work with a woman who has around 10 or 15 pounds to lose, there appears to be this gravitational pull back towards health. The body can pretty much correct itself fairly easily when you have 10 to 15 pounds to lose if you're doing the right things. If you're just flat out doing the wrong things, then no, you're not going to see results.

These are the type of people who can typically just cut back on sugar and cut out the carbs or cut out eating bad foods. They increase their exercise a little bit. If they are consistent with that approach long enough, then they can lose that weight fairly quickly. It works out great, and it's what most people do their entire life.

They gain 10 pounds and they can lose it. They gain 10 pounds again and they can lose it. They gain 10 pounds once more and then maybe they end up creeping up to 15 pounds, then they lose it. This is how a lot of women spend their lives, just going back and forth between this 10 and 15 pounds of excess weight, which is usually fine. You're not necessarily in a zone of bad health when you're in that range. However, if you don't correct the problem at 15 pounds, then things very, very quickly start to escalate.

This is the point where women just seem to feel like they woke up one day and have no idea what happened. They were always able to lose the weight between the 10- and 15-pound range. And they think it's going to be the same situation when they get to 20, 25, or 40 pounds. They think they can just try the various diets that you see in the magazines: "The Seven Tips for Flat Abs Before Summer," "Eat This One Food and Lose Weight in a Week," or "Drink This Detox Elixir and Lose Three Pounds Tomorrow" and the many YouTube videos with the at-home exercises. But what they don't realize is that all of those things only work on the people who typically have less than 10 to 15 pounds to lose. They don't understand this concept that your body is storing fat at a rapid pace because there is a deeper, underlying issue that's not being addressed, and it's not going to be fixed by doing the latest fad or body hack.

When you have more than 15 pounds to lose, the systems inside the body are severely out of balance and begin to work against you. This is why traditional diets and exercises no longer work for you. And weight loss is much more difficult after you've gone past the tipping point. Seemingly, everything you do is in vain. You don't understand because you look at your friend who is eating the same exact thing as you or who never works out but is not gaining any weight. "Why am I gaining all this weight and she's not?" It's because you've gotten gone past the body tipping point!

Along with weight becoming more difficult to lose, the more overweight you are, the extra pounds also have the potential to cause major health issues. Similarly, the more you lose, the more you decrease your risk for disease. Victor Stevens, Ph.D., a Kaiser Permanente researcher in a weight loss study, found that losing as little as five pounds can reduce the risk of developing high blood pressure by 20 percent. If just losing five pounds can have such a positive impact on your health, imagine what losing 20, 30, or 50 pounds could do for you.

Another reason you want to address this problem now rather than later is that it's only going to get worse and worse each year or the longer you wait to try to turn this around. Your body will continue to pack on weight year after year, but not necessarily because you are getting older or because you are eating too much or not exercising enough. It's because fat cells in your body secrete inflammatory chemicals that block your ability to burn fat. It's a Catch-22! Having excess inflammation in the body keeps you from being able to lose weight.

The good news is that the 3X Program will help you bring your body back towards the other side of the teeter totter where you can lose the weight, improve your health, and get your body back to normal.

The following testimonial is from my client Julie G., who struggled with joint inflammation and excess weight.

After being diagnosed in 2012 with Psoriatic Arthritis, I struggled with my weight because being active became difficult and painful. My wonderful friend James recommended that I try a new program called 3X Weight Loss.

When I began, I was the heaviest I had ever been in my life. I stand at 5'4" and at the time, I weighed 167 pounds. After the program, in just three months, I lost 48 pounds and went from a size 14 to a size 2.

But I did not do 3X Weight Loss to look cute in clothes. With Laura's help, I learned all about how my body processes food and how to bring the inflammation down in my joints, which has helped with my arthritis and my overall quality of life. Now, I play tennis twice a week, I have so much energy, my thinking is clearer, my arthritis is much more manageable and I'm thriving in my career. If it had not been for Laura and this life-changing program, I would not be where I am today.

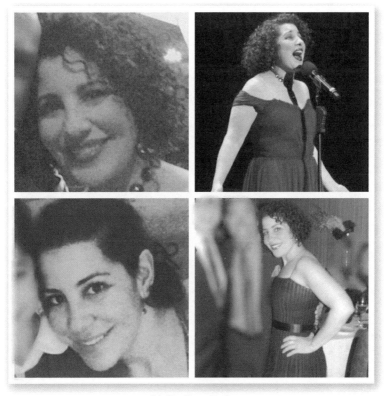

It's Not Your Fault

The fact that you haven't been able to get desired results in the past does not mean you are the problem. The reason diet and exercise programs have failed you is that you most likely focused on trying to fix the symptom instead of the cause. **You can do this.** You just need the right program and the right person to explain it to you.

I learned the hard way that the world of dieting is full of scams, lies, and empty promises. It's so easy to fall for gimmicks that tell you to just take a magic pill or that you can somehow still lose weight without giving up your favorite foods. There is so much false information out there about weight loss and it can all be very overwhelming and confusing to know exactly what steps to take that will actually get results.

In fact, most diet and exercise programs are actually telling you to do the exact opposite of what you should, which is why it's so hard to lose weight. So believe me when I say that I get it. I know exactly where you're at. I'll bet you'll be as shocked as I was when you realize that by working with your body, instead of against it, it's actually a very simple process.

When you take the correct approach (the forthcoming information that I will teach you), you can reset your metabolism to burn deep into your fat stores at its most efficient rate. This will allow you to lose weight three times faster and keep it off for good. This is where it gets exciting!

Once you get into this fat burning state, everything you do burns fat. You don't even have to think about it anymore. You won't be constantly wondering what you should do to lose weight. You will be burning fat with everything you do, whether you're sitting at your desk answering emails, or driving in your car on the way to work. Your body will constantly be burning fat. You will even be burning fat in your sleep!

If you follow the protocol that I lay out for you in this book, you can get into and stay in a healthy fat-burning mode and win the weight loss game once and for all.

I want to introduce you to my friend Hilda, who has lost 90 pounds to date on this program. Here is her story.

All my life I have struggled with my weight. I tried Venus De Milo at age 15, Redax at age 17, Jenny Craig and jogging three miles a day at 25 years old. I did Atkins diet at 26. I had a personal trainer at 27. I had liposuction done at 30. And at 40 I tried Lindora.

I was invited to Weight Watchers, Kickboxing, Zumba, Boot Camp, and even did a popular shake diet. I asked myself, how could I live on powder? No way, I loved food! I was so tired of always trying the next diet fad and exercise trend. I would lose some weight, but I always gained it all back and then some.

I went from 255 to 300 pounds and I didn't know what to do about stopping this miserable cycle. I was taking 20 milligrams of Lisinopril daily for high blood pressure, and my glucose levels were at 101. I was headed toward complete health destruction and couldn't seem to reverse this vicious cycle.

By the grace of God, my sister Patty showed me a picture of a friend on Facebook who had lost 40 pounds at the time but has now lost 60 pounds and who has kept it off for two years following the 3X Program. So I took a leap of faith.

I started the program in August 2015 at the age of 51, and in the first two months I lost 27 pounds, which was astounding. To date, I have lost more than 85 pounds without exercise. It's amazing how I have also lost the brain frog and much of the fatigue I used to experience. In addition, my high blood pressure normalized, and I no longer have signs of pre-diabetes.

My doctor was floored and asked me what I was doing because all the signs of inflammation were gone. He gave me kudos and told me to keep it up. And I knew I would because this lifestyle was so easy to maintain.

My ultimate goal was to lose 100 pounds. I no longer have a doubt I will reach my goal or maybe even exceed it. Once I hit the 100 mark, I will make it my mission to fly out to Utah to thank the founder of this program in person, my friend Laura Sales. Without the creation of her program, I don't know where I would be or if I would even be here to tell you my story.

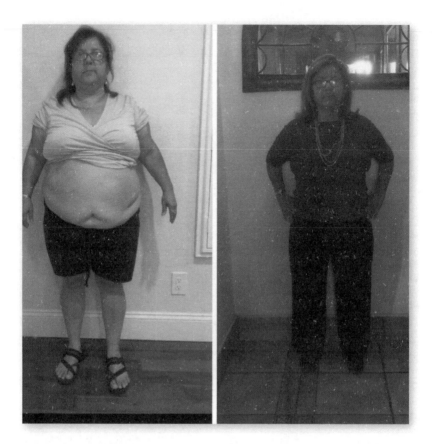

That's just one of many of my client success stories. Personally, it makes me feel so good to know that I'm helping so many women on deeper levels than just losing excess weight. As we proceed throughout the book, keep Hilda's story in mind. If she could do it with 100 pounds to lose, you can do it too!

IS 3X WEIGHT LOSS FOR ME?

You're following closely so far and even felt a glimmer of hope after reading Hilda's story. But you're probably still thinking, "How do I know 3X Weight Loss will work for me?" This is one of the most frequent questions I am asked. The truth is that 3X Weight Loss wasn't created for women who have an easy time losing weight (although it will still work for them). It is geared towards women who have a completely stalled metabolism from years of crash dieting and exercising or from having too much stress and poor hormonal health.

With that said, 3X Weight Loss has consistently produced amazing results for thousands of women all around the world. **It does not matter what your situation is; this program will work for you.** In fact, I have not yet met a woman who couldn't be helped with this approach. Whether a mother of five or none. Whether having a thyroid condition or slow metabolism. The program is even effective through menopause. So don't worry, you will reach your goal weight with 3X Weight Loss no matter how much you have to lose or what your situation is.

You are the ideal candidate for this program if you've experienced any of the following:

- You've failed miserably at reaching your weight-loss goal in the past.
- You're currently on a diet or exercise program but aren't seeing results.
- You can easily lose weight but keeping it off seems impossible.
- You're actually scared to try another diet because the thought of it not working is your biggest fear.
- If you have severe sugar cravings, food addictions, food intolerances, gut issues, or hormonal problems.
- If you aren't getting results with exercise, have no time to exercise or can't exercise because of some physical condition.

In other words, if you feel that you need a complete metabolism makeover, this program is for you because that is exactly what it is.

Here is another success story from my client Catherine, who finally found a healthy way to lose her troublesome excess weight through 3X:

I am 56 years old, way past menopause, and have been carrying around a lot of extra weight ever since I had my third child twenty-seven years ago. That was a very stressful birth, and somehow the weight never came off like it had with my first two children. On the contrary, I just gained more and more weight, even though I've always been active and eaten healthy.

A few years ago, I ballooned up to the highest I'd ever been, and I put myself on a strict low-calorie, no-sugar, 30-minutes-of-exercise-a-day-and-lots-of-water diet. It took me six months to lose 20 pounds, and each pound was grueling and painful. I couldn't keep up the torture, and so I stopped the diet and in the next year I gained it all back. Then my husband died, and I gave up any pretense of taking care of myself and gained another ten pounds in a few months.

None of my clothes fit and I was feeling awful physically, with aches and pains in every part of my body. My kids were urging me to do something for my health. They didn't want to lose both parents. Then a friend told me about 3X Weight Loss. I was worried at first, because so many diets I'd seen out there required starving yourself (which I couldn't do), taking hormones (which I knew would be terrible for my health), or eating pre-packaged meals which had gluten or other foods that I was allergic to. But my friend said it was nothing like that, so I tried it, and she was right; it wasn't.

3X is a very healthy program based on taking all the things that are unhealthy out of your diet and only eating healthy things and taking supplements that stem the cravings. As soon as I got on the program, I immediately felt better, and I lost two pounds in the first day. As the days went on, I kept losing and kept feeling better. It was much easier than the diet I put myself on a few years ago, and it was painless, and I really didn't experience many cravings.

Now I've been on the program for six months and I've lost more than 50 lbs and am continuing to lose. I am feeling healthy, and I didn't get any of the colds or flus that were going around in the winter months. I am fitting into normal-sized clothes and am officially not obese per my BMI, and I look younger and prettier.

I really appreciate all the work Laura Sales put into making the program. It has made it possible for me to keep my New Year's resolution.

–Catherine W.

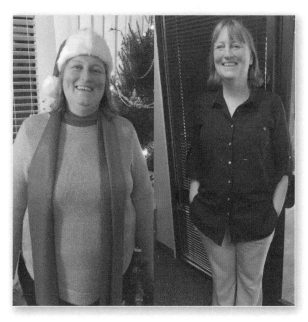

CHAPTER 2

THE CALORIE MYTH

Have you ever known someone who could eat whatever they wanted and not gain weight? Perhaps you experienced a time in your life when it didn't matter what you ate or how little you exercised and you were still in great shape. We can all rattle off names of friends or family who were a size four or six on their wedding day and by the time they had two or three kids or after they reached their late thirties, they had gained thirty or forty pounds. And no matter how much they dieted or exercised, the stubborn pounds just wouldn't budge. I don't know about you, but I have met many women who have told me, "I am eating less than I did when I was in college and I'm twenty-five pounds heavier!" The question is, how could this be if weight loss is all about calories in vs. calories out? Aha!

When it comes to weight loss, a large portion of our population, including most conventional doctors and dieticians, have it all wrong. We have basically all been brainwashed to believe that weight loss is a simple matter of calories in versus calories out. That in order to lose weight, all we have to do is reduce the number of calories we consume and increase the number of calories we burn through exercise.

To the people who subscribe to this theory, a calorie is just a calorie. It doesn't matter if the calories come from soda, candy, or a cup of spinach; they believe that when it comes to weight loss, all calories are created equal. According to this theory, you could eat pizza and ice cream (as long as you only had a certain number of calories) then you could go to the gym and run on the treadmill for hours to "burn it all off." Girl, let me just tell you that this theory has taken us down a very dark tunnel that leads to diet and exercise HELL.

If this were actually true, we'd all be at our ideal body weight, but that's hardly the case. Instead, we are underfed, undernourished, overworked, and overweight. The calorie method is the biggest diet lie that's ever been told.

One pound of fat is 3500 calories. Just reduce your daily caloric intake by 500 calories and after a week, you'll lose one pound of fat. If you want to lose two pounds a week, just go to the gym every day and burn more calories! Sounds too good to be true, right? That's because it is. While it's true that excess calories of the *wrong* foods lead to weight gain, different foods have drastically different effects on our digestion, our metabolism and the way our bodies burn fuel for energy and store body fat.

I am not entirely saying that calories don't matter because in some manner they do. However, to say that our body metabolizes table sugar the same as spinach would be a flat-out lie. Calories do play a small role in weight loss, but not in the traditional way we've all grown accustomed to (calories in versus out).

In this section, I want to hit home on how weight loss is not about calories in versus calories out or eating less and exercising more. I'll explain how flawed the theory is and how we've all been duped to believe something that is scientifically not true.

There are major misconceptions about calories, fat loss, and health, some of which are rooted in truth but have been oversimplified to the point that people have fallen into the trap of thinking all calories are created equal in relation to fat loss. This is not the case. This common misconception has caused people to think it's okay to consume empty calories as long as they stay within a specific calorie range or as long as they go to the gym to make up for it. The "calorie is a calorie" myth is out-of-date, and this old way of thinking is why so many women are struggling to lose weight.

Can you imagine using an old computer from the 1970s? How about using a phone, VCR, or tape player from the 1980s? What about a television from 50 years ago? You'd laugh at the idea of using outdated technology! Why not use that the same approach with your health and ditch the obsolete eating approaches that are 50 years old and scientifically disproven?

Unfortunately, medical doctors, old-school dieticians, the U.S. government, and food manufacturers are to this day promoting the outdated theory that all calories are created equal. Understandably, the food industry has a lot to gain by people subscribing to this way of thinking. In fact, the food industry has made billions of dollars off the calorie theory with their pre-packaged, low-fat diet foods that have all but replaced real food. In my opinion, this is probably why they refuse to admit otherwise even though new scientific research has proven that it is not the most effective means to lose weight.

The longstanding belief that all you have to do is burn more calories than you consume to lose weight is false. If we want to quit struggling with weight loss, we have to change the way we think about calories in vs. calories out. Statistically, we're getting fatter every decade (including our children) regardless of how little we eat and how much exercise we do, and we aren't going to lose weight and get healthy until we stop relying on false, outdated information.

THE BIGGEST DIET LIE: ALL CALORIES ARE CREATED EQUAL

Calories in versus calories out: Sounds nice and simple, just the way we like it. Simple is great when you're trying to learn a new computer program, but overly simple can be extremely dangerous to your health.

This whole theory came about because scientists discovered that in an isolated system, like in a laboratory setting, 500 calories of table sugar is the same as 500 calories of cauliflower. When tested, the 500 calories of sugar and 500 calories of cauliflower released identical amounts of energy. But when scientists applied this theory in the real world, they must have forgotten the fact that we are not isolated subjects in a laboratory; We are humans. We are complex living, breathing, organisms.

When you eat 500 calories of straight sugar, the body is going to digest and process it very differently than if you ate 500 calories of cauliflower. So, the "isolated system" experiment and "a calorie is just a calorie" outcome becomes entirely inapplicable when you relate it to humans.

Imagine for a moment that you're a ninth grader again and you're studying nutrition. Your teacher has two large bowls in the front of the classroom. One bowl is filled with a mixture of white flour and sugar. The other bowl is filled with a colorful array of freshly picked vegetables from a garden. Your teacher asks the class, "Do these two bowls have the same effect on your body nutritionally?" Of course, the class's response is a unanimous "NO!" Intuitively, most reasonable adults know that equal caloric amounts of sugar and white flour are not the same as vegetables. But for some reason, a lot of us prefer to pretend they're the same so that we can have our cake and eat it too.

Let me be completely clear here: Your body does burn calories. However, the type of calories you consume makes all the difference when it comes to how your body either stores fat or burns it. It certainly would be nice if it were as simple as counting calories. Then, reducing the number of calories we consume and increasing our level of exercise would mean that fat would melt off effortlessly. And anyone who could do basic addition and subtraction could have an amazing figure. But that's not the case, now is it? And the current obesity epidemic makes that very clear.

Like everyone else, I'd love to believe that cake and salmon are nutritionally similar and all that matters are their caloric amounts. In reality, though, cake and salmon are not created equal. Metabolically speaking, they have very different fates once they enter our bodies. If you were to live off 1800 calories a day from boxed cake for two weeks, it would have a very different effect than if you lived off 1800 calories a day of Alaskan wild-caught salmon for two weeks.

Can you now understand how a calorie is not just a calorie?

WEIGHT LOSS IS NOT THE SAME AS FAT LOSS

The calories-in-versus-calories-out theory has, at best, limited short-term workability. You may have experienced a time when following the calorie method actually worked for you. However, I can bet, especially since you are reading this book, that you are no longer able to get results with it despite continuing to eat less and exercise more. Am I right? I can also pretty much guarantee that the weight you lost (if any) was mostly water weight and muscle. Believe it or not, while you thought you were doing something good for your body by taking this approach, you were actually harming your metabolism and made it that much harder for you to lose actual body fat (this goes for those other diet programs too).

When we want to see the number on the scale go down, we typically think to ourselves, "I want to lose weight," but that's too general. Our thought process should instead be focused on losing body fat while retaining or gaining muscle mass.

Studies have shown that the *type* of foods we eat can affect whether we lose unwanted fat or precious muscle, which we absolutely want to keep. So in order to be successful, we must pay attention to the nutrient composition of the foods we eat.

When it comes to the number on the scale, losing "weight" doesn't tell the whole story. The real question you should be asking when you notice you've lost weight is, "What kind of weight did I lose? Was it lean muscle mass or was it body fat?" It is also very important to know if you are losing body fat while gaining muscle. Is your weight loss based on an empty-calorie, sugar-laden diet that's devoid of nutrients, or are you eating nutritious foods that are improving your health during the weight loss process?

The type of food you eat has a **direct** impact on weight loss and your health. When you consume 300 calories of raw spinach, it will have very different metabolic effects than 300 calories of pizza. That's because spinach is chock full of vitamins A, C, E, K, B2, B6, folate, iron, calcium, potassium, zinc, manganese, and copper. It's also a good source of dietary fiber, protein, and choline. Pizza, on the other hand, is devoid of nutrients and does nothing to build muscle or a healthy immune system. The nutrients (or lack thereof) in the foods we eat are the factors that count when it comes to losing and gaining body fat.

IS LOSING WEIGHT QUICKLY UNSAFE?

Understanding the impact of weight loss on your health may spark you to want to lose as much weight as possible, as quickly as possible. That is OK, though we often hear otherwise. Experts say that it's not safe to lose more than one to two pounds per week because they are operating off the seriously flawed, old-school method of calories in versus calories out.

Based on the definition of a calorie being "a unit of energy," they came up with the fact that to produce energy the body burns calories. It was then determined that 3,500 calories equaled a pound of fat, so in order to lose one pound per week, you would have to create a deficit of 3,500 calories per week (-500 calories per day). If you wanted to lose two pounds in a week, you'd have a 7,000-calorie deficit (-1000 per day).

The average female burns 1,500 calories per day at rest. So if you do the math, in order to maintain her current weight she could consume 1,500 calories per day and would not gain weight. If she wanted to lose one pound per week, she would have to reduce her calories by 500 per day, which would mean she could consume 1,000 calories per day. Or she could eat 1,250 calories as long as she exercised and burned 250 calories.

Keeping up with this math, if she wanted to lose two pounds per week, which would be 7,000 calories per week, she would technically have to reduce her calories by 1,000 per day which means she could only eat 500 calories per day. That is starvation. Or she could eat 1,000 calories if she went to the gym and burned 500 calories every single day. Do you know how many hours you would have to run on the treadmill to burn 500 calories? Two and a half hours. So in this scenario, this woman is pretty much starving every day and has to go to the gym and run for two and a half hours. How miserable!

Based on this theory, if you wanted to lose more than two pounds per week, you would have to eat 0 calories per day and then go to the gym and burn a bunch of calories. This approach is neither safe nor recommended. And this is why they all say it's not safe to lose more than 1-2 pounds per week.

I can confidently tell you, **you can lose more than one to two pounds per week and when you do it the right way without**

relying on calorie restrictions, starving, or exercising, then it is absolutely safe. What's NOT safe is carrying around 10, 20, 30, 40, or 50+ pounds of toxic body fat that is putting a serious toll on your health. Losing the weight is not only safe but vital.

By the way, if you follow the protocol I lay out for you in the upcoming pages, you will see that you can lose a lot more than 1-2 pounds per week. The average weight loss without restricting calories or requiring exercise is 26.7 pounds in 60 days. So it would take you a lot less than six months. This is why the program is called 3X Weight Loss. We lose weight 3X faster and keep it off without starving, cravings, or willpower!

EMPTY CALORIES MAKE YOU FEEL EMPTY

In order to be successful though, you can't feel hungry all the time! If you've ever been on a restricted-calorie diet, you've probably had difficulty sticking to it. Not only were the results either too slow or not there at all, but the continual feeling of deprivation and starvation makes it very hard to stay committed long enough to reach your goal.

The reason you may have felt hungry and deprived on other diets is because most low-calorie diet foods are devoid of essential vitamins, minerals, and healthy fats and believe it or not, are usually filled with flavor additivities and sugar! Both flavor enhancers and sugar cause food addictions, never leaving you full or satisfied and always making you more and more hungry.

Have you ever noticed that you could eat an entire tub of ice cream or a whole box of cookies or a full bag of chips, but when it comes to eating salad or fruit you tend to only eat a regular portion before you feel satisfied? I bet you've never binged on a bowl of spinach. This is because eating wholesome food sends signals to your brain that you are actually full and satisfied. Conversely, when bad foods are consumed, they do not send the same signals to our body as whole food, regardless of whether they have the same number of calories in them.

Eating a whole box of processed cookies is not the same as consuming an equal number of calories in raw vegetables. You could eat 1,000 calories of cookies easily, but it's going to be a lot harder to consume 1,000 calories of raw vegetables.

Because of the volume of all those vegetables, your stomach would send a message to your brain that you were full. Unlike a high-sugar meal, the vegetables would not trigger the addiction-reward center in your brain. Ever heard of someone being "addicted" to vegetables? Sugar or soda, yes, but not veggies! You would also enjoy the numerous metabolism-boosting benefits of eating vegetables: lowered cholesterol, detoxification, and reduced inflammation. Let us not forget that many of the vitamins in vegetables help balance hormones and protect the body against cancer and heart disease. What I'm hopefully making crystal clear is that **all calories are NOT created equal.**

To put things into perspective, it's important to understand that some calories (think sugar) are addictive. Some calories are fattening. And others have properties that will actually boost your metabolism. Why? It's because food contains so much more than calories. It contains information. Every bite you put into your mouth comes with a complete set of biological instructions to your body. It either promotes health or it increases the risk of disease. So what will it be, a dozen of your favorite packaged cookies, or a steak and a salad for dinner?

When you eat empty calories, you're still hungry because your body did not get any nutrients out of the food. In contrast, when you eat a meal that's full of healthy proteins, carbohydrates (from vegetables) and fats (think olive, avocado, or coconut oil), you're likely to eat much fewer calories because these foods actually help to reduce appetite. Unlike simple carbohydrates, which don't suppress hunger, foods full of macronutrients activate leptin, the hormone that decreases appetite and suppresses ghrelin, the hormone that increases the appetite. The best thing is to get our calories from foods that burn fat, produce satiation, increase immunity, decrease inflammation, and help protect our bodies against disease.

Bottom line: Saying that being overweight is solely caused by too many calories does not paint the whole picture because it says nothing about the actual causes behind weight gain. This drastic oversimplification doesn't take into account the fact that different foods have varying metabolic pathways. It also doesn't account for the different effects food has on our hormones and brain chemistry. To say a calorie is a calorie is outdated and we have to stop believing this theory if we want to experience lasting weight loss. Once you get past the calorie-is-a-calorie myth, then and only then will you realize that you can actually eat food, eat fat, and NOT rely on willpower—yet still lose weight.

In order to not jump into old (bad) habits, we needed to establish the foundation of why you weren't losing weight and how so much of the available information is incorrect. Now that you have a solid understanding of this, we'll jump into explaining how your body actually loses weight.

CHAPTER 3

HOW WEIGHT LOSS REALLY WORKS

Here is how weight loss really works. Your body has two sources of energy that it can use to function. It can get energy from either glucose (which is sugar) or it can get energy from stored fat.

Most people who are trying to lose weight are only burning glucose and rarely, if ever, tap into stored fat. They will go on a diet and start an exercise program, but all they lose is the initial water weight (thinking that it's actually fat but it's not) and then they hit a plateau, so they try the next diet, and then the next, and eventually get to a point where "nothing seems to work." They wonder why they can never reach their ideal weight. This is because they are only burning sugar and not burning real fat.

Logically, if your objective is fat loss, then you would want your body to use up stored fat as energy instead of using glucose. How else do you think your fat cells are going to disappear? They get "burned" and melt away when the body uses them for energy, which results in losing weight.

The problem is that the body *prefers* to use glucose for energy. It doesn't want to use up fat because it is the body's "backup supply" of fuel. The storing of excess fat is actually a survival mechanism that is built into our genetic code. The only way our body will tap into fat stores and burn fat instead of glucose is if there *is no glucose to be used*. It will always choose glucose first and factually cannot burn fat when it is present.

So what is glucose and where does it come from? Glucose is another word for sugar and it comes from the food that you eat. You don't have to eat white table sugar to be consuming glucose. All food eventually gets broken down into varying amounts of glucoses (except fat). Glucose stimulates the fat storage hormone insulin. Insulin's job is to take glucose out of the blood stream and into the cells. If there is too much sugar in the bloodstream resulting from eating high glucose- type foods, everything will be stored in the fat cells.

So how do you provide an environment within your body where it has no choice but to use fat for energy? The key is to only eat foods that result in little to no stimulus of insulin. because that way, your body will have to tap into your fat reserves to get the energy it needs. That is the simple and fundamental way your body burns fat.

Now, this may or may not be shocking information to you. I am certainly not the first one to have made these statements. All low-carb diets such as Atkins, Ketosis, and South Beach are based on these principles, and regardless of the criticism they receive, these approaches *are* very effective at burning fat. The "problem" with these programs is that they are solely focused on burning fat without regard for overall health, which is great for weight loss, but not so great for long-term vitality.

The bottom line is this: The body can be forced to lose weight with deprivation diets (low calorie), by extreme exercise routines or with no-carb diets, or it can do it naturally, which is the healthier way that doesn't require either of those things. That is where the 3X program comes in.

So how exactly does 3X Weight Loss work? 3X Weight Loss is based on an x-factor that is rarely talked about: homeostasis. Homeostasis simply means balance. It refers to the ability of the body to seek and maintain a condition of stability within its internal environment when dealing with external changes. Or, in plain English, it means getting your body back to normal.

Phase 1 of 3X Weight Loss is a metabolism-reset program that focuses on healing the body and bringing it back toward a state of balance. During this phase, we focus on giving your body the right nutrients to feel safe in releasing fat and establishing the core principles of a healthy lifestyle so that you develop habits that turn into a normal daily routine.

HOW IS 3X WEIGHT LOSS DIFFERENT?

Instead of being just another unrealistic, short-term diet, 3X Weight Loss helps to establish healthy lifestyle habits that reset your metabolism, bringing it back into a state of balance. This approach will not only drastically improve your health, but will also be the catalyst to lose weight and keep it off for good.

We do this by correcting the underlying issues within your metabolism and working with your body to get it back into a state of homeostasis. It's not a "cleanse" or a detox program, nor a 30-day challenge, nor a fad. It's different from every other program out there because instead of addressing the symptom of having excess weight, it addresses the cause.

The second way this program is different is that it puts you in control by teaching you how weight loss works. Because the truth is—drum roll please—if losing weight and keeping it off is something you really want, you need to understand how your body works. At least a little bit! Trust me when I say that this point alone is the missing link to all other programs and is the key to losing weight and keeping it off for good.

Think back to all the diets you tried in the past. Did you ever really know why you were being told reduce your calories and eat low fat? Or why you were being told to do 30 minutes of cardio three to five times per week? Probably not, and this is why dieting can be so frustrating! Without knowing *why* you are doing what you are doing, you'll always be at the mercy of whatever diet or weight-loss program has better marketing. And you'll never get the long-term results you are looking for. So you need to decide if you want to take a little bit of time now to learn how your body works, or if you are going to spend the rest of your life dieting.

Now we are going to get into the technical side of things. I promise to make it fun and interesting, and above all else, easy to understand! Please put on your schoolgirl hat and let's get through this next section together and carefully, because everything I am going to discuss is absolutely crucial to your success on this program.

WHAT IS HOMEOSTASIS?

The first process we'll review is called "homeostasis." Your body is constantly trying to achieve a state of balance. As an example, when you get too hot, your body works to cool itself down by sweating. When you get too cold, your body heats up to keep you warm. When you have excess fat, your fat cells tell your brain you have enough stored energy so it can reduce hunger and start burning fat. Well, this is what's *supposed* to happen but only when your body is balanced and working correctly.

If you eat more calories, your body will burn more calories. If you eat fewer calories, your body will burn fewer calories (another reason why calories in versus calories out makes no sense). Get the point? You see, your body is constantly working to achieve this ideal state of balance. You shouldn't have to *try* to lose weight. Your body already knows what to do and believe it or not, it wants to be at a healthy weight.

HOMEOSTASIS

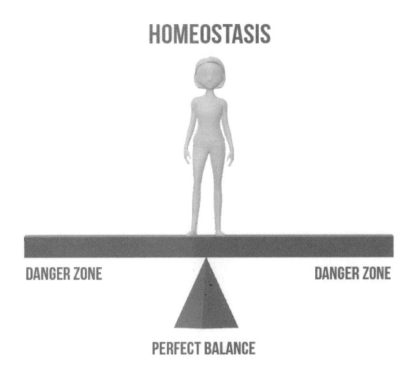

DANGER ZONE   DANGER ZONE

PERFECT BALANCE

Whether or not your body can maintain an ideal state of balance depends upon whether its balancing mechanism is functioning. Due to a number of factors such as stress, lack of sleep, wrong types of exercise, wrong types of food, nutritional deficiencies, and toxins, the body gets thrown out of balance. As hard as it works to come back to balance on its own, usually since it's overburdened and undernourished, it is unable to and this is when a person starts to go further away from homeostasis, begins to gain weight, and begins to decline in health.

The key to great health and rapid, natural weight loss is to work with your body to achieve this ideal state of balance. That is what the 3X Weight Loss Program does and it's the reason that on this program, you will get three times better results than others. My focus is to work with your body to get it to do what it is naturally meant to do.

Below is a testimonial that illustrates how 3X has changed lives by simply understanding the body's needs and giving it nutrients it requires.

The 3X Weight Loss Program has been the best program for my clients and myself. As a wellness coach and nutritional consultant, I was actually very sad that I could not help my clients with Hashimoto's and other autoimmune diseases lose those pesky pounds because I COULD NOT HELP MYSELF lose them.

When you have a thyroid issue, it makes weight loss virtually impossible. Add menopause and other metabolism killers like yo-yo dieting and you have a real recipe to not only keep on the pounds, literally, your body REFUSING to let them go, but also watching the scale creep up year after year.

I was devastated for my clients and feeling like a fraud as a coach. Then along came a prior client who changed my life both physically and professionally. She told me about the 3X Program and it immediately clicked as the right thing to do. I started it immediately.

The thing that spoke to me the most was Laura emphatically claiming that "this program works on everyone," meaning exactly what I was looking for was found!!

The 3X Weight Loss Program works beautifully for peri- and post-menopausal women, women with Hashimoto's, and other thyroid/hormone issues. It actually seems to REPAIR the crashed metabolism that so many of my clients suffered from because of years of diets that starve you and confuse the body into thinking it must hold onto every calorie. It actually handles that for every client I have put on it.

For myself, I have lost over 13 pounds and still counting. I went from a size 8/9 pant and skirt to a size 4/6. My skin looks more toned even though I only recently added exercise back in. I had to lower my thyroid meds because my thyroid actually started DOING ITS JOB!!!!

The real science behind this program is that it restores homeostasis and that means it brings your body back to its true state—the state that it was meant to be in. When that is restored, your body will work the way it is supposed to.

On top of that, this is a complete anti-inflammation diet— that is how my thyroid started to work. It worked on reducing the inflammation (which is the true underlying reason for Autoimmune Disease flare-ups, etc.). My clients with diabetes, high blood pressure etc. all report drops in their once very scary numbers.

ALL of my clients report feeling better and having increased energy, better sleep, and moods. One husband of a client actually called to thank me "for giving him his lovely wife back." She is "like a new person."

This is the perfect plan for people who have tried everything, can't lose the weight, and/or fight food cravings that cave them in and make them fall off the wagon diet after diet after diet. That is partly because this is NOT a diet but a real-life, workable lifestyle program to feel good, look good, and feel great—for GOOD!

My 15 or so clients and I could not be happier. The program, the supplements and the support are all of what make the difference. I could not be happier personally or professionally.

The 3X Program is your last diet.

-Nancy M.

So where do you begin? It all starts with your metabolism. Adjusting your lifestyle so that your metabolism can reach an ideal state of homeostasis is the first step to achieving long lasting health and weight-loss results.

RESETTING YOUR METABOLISM

A lot of people talk about the word "metabolism," but rarely does anyone define it or break it down to show you what it looks like, how it runs, and what it needs to function optimally.

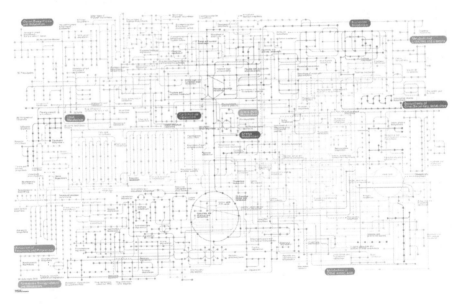

Source: www.harvardmagazine.com

Above is a picture of a human body metabolism. Amazing, right?! Every single line you see in that image is a process that has to take place in order for you to stay alive and be healthy.

Your metabolism is responsible for every single function in your entire body. It is not just about how many calories you burn and how fast or slowly you lose weight. A few of the vital, everyday functions of your metabolism are to keep your heart beating, to keep your lungs breathing, and maintaining the circulation of your blood.

In order to find out exactly what metabolism had to do with weight loss and overall health, I studied the research done by Dr. Bruce Ames, a professor of biochemistry and molecular biology at the University of California, Berkeley. He has done extensive research regarding the influence of nutrition on the metabolism and is a recipient of the National Medal of Science from President Bill Clinton, has published more than 550 papers, and is one of the most-cited scientists across all fields.

In his research, he found that over 50 enzymes are completely dependent upon daily intake of adequate amounts of vitamins, minerals, and essential fatty acids. Enzymes are the "worker bees" and are the ones responsible for getting the job done within our metabolism. They are the sparks that start the essential chemical reactions our bodies need to live. They are necessary for digesting food, stimulating the brain, providing cellular energy, and repairing all tissues, organs, and cells.

It has been found that there are over 40 essential nutrients that these enzymes need to carry out their daily duties. "Essential" means that our bodies cannot make these nutrients on their own and so they must be obtained from our diet. Without consistent, adequate levels of these nutrients every day, it is impossible for the body's enzymes to begin their work and for humans to experience vital health and optimal metabolism. This puts a new perspective on nutrition and, in my opinion, gives new meaning to what the purpose of food is!

The real purpose of food is to nourish the body so that it can run optimally. Getting enough of vitamins and minerals every day is essential to not only a high-functioning metabolism, but these can also be the vital difference between optimum health and the simple absence of an illness. And there is a vast difference between these two extremes.

Because of the lack of nutrients that most of the food we consume contains, it is not surprising that most people in the world are deficient in at least one of the 40 vitamins, minerals, and other essential nutrients necessary daily for minimal survival. Because the human body was created with a natural ability to adapt to amazing variables and still survive, we see that most women today experience life not in a state of vital health, but fluctuating on the continuum of health between chronic disease and "not sick."

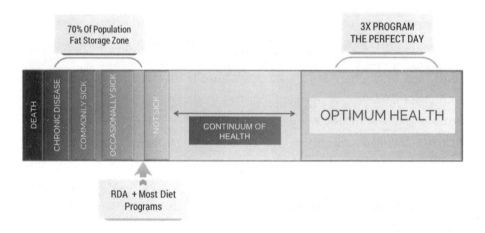

Source: www.3xweightloss.com

People on the left side of the continuum of health are shockingly deficient in essential nutrients. These are crucial to controlling blood sugar levels, stress responses, conversion of foods into usable forms that can actually nourish the body, and controlling every enzyme reaction needed for our metabolism to work.

As a nation, Americans are overfed and yet, undernourished and chronically stressed. This chronic state of deficiency results in a downshifting of the metabolism to attempt to spare what nutrient resources are remaining. In most cases, this manifests as mental sluggishness, poor digestion, daytime fatigue, poor sleep, chronic aches and pain due to inflammation, and cravings that are not satisfied by food. Does any of this sound familiar?

As the brain signals the body to input more nutrients to try to satisfy these vital deficiencies and people answer these signals with low-nutrient convenience foods high in sugar, starch, vegetable oils, chemical additives, and stimulants, the metabolism continues to down-regulate and disease breeds at a faster rate. Put simply, when you feel hungry, it is critical to feed your body with foods that will nourish it. Otherwise, there is no purpose to what you are ingesting and you will be harming your body in one way or another. Remember, a calorie is no longer just a calorie when you think in terms of optimal nutrition needed for your body to be healthy.

Question for you: Now that you know your metabolism requires 40 essential nutrients to perform optimally, do you think eating pizza (or other low-quality food), even though you don't go over a certain number of calories, is going to give your metabolism the nutrients that it needs to run fast and efficiently?

Great job on answering, "No." Each complex action that is performed by your metabolism requires essential vitamins, minerals, fatty acids and amino acids in order to function. It does not require a certain number of calories. This is, again, why the calories-in-versus-calories-out theory of weight loss is **complete nonsense**.

The next question is then, what are these micronutrients and how much of them do you need? Here is a list of the essential micronutrients by Dr. Bruce Ames needed by your metabolism daily.

Biotin	Calcium	Linolenic Acid/DHA
Folate	Chloride	(Omega-3)
Niacin	Chromium	Linoleic acid (Omega-6)
Pantothenate	Choline	Isoleucine (Amino Acid)
Riboflavin	Cobalt	Leucine (Amino Acid)
Thiamine	Copper	Lysine (Amino Acid)
Vitamin A	Histidine (Amino Acid)	Methionine (Amino Acid)
Vitamin B6	Iodide	Phenylalanine (Amino Acid)
Vitamin B12	Iron	Threonine (Amino Acid)
Vitamin C	Magnesium	Tryptophan (Amino Acid)
Vitamin E	Manganese	Valine (Amino Acid)
Vitamin K	Molybdenum	Zinc
Selenium	Phosphorus	
Potassium	Sodium	

Source: Bruce Ames - Vitamin and Mineral Inadequacy Accelerates Aging-Associated Diseases at Montana State University https://www.youtube.com/watch?v=VmvG4ur7HnU

You do not need to get these micronutrients every once in a while. You need to get them every day, at *least* twice a day, to be exact.

That means that the salad you had for lunch three days ago that you thought was going to give you your nutritional requirements for the week is long gone. And that green smoothie you might have had for breakfast is used up by mid-afternoon. Dr. Ames says that even if you are a little bit deficient in one of these micronutrients, you're going to pay a price. He says at a minimum, it's going to age you faster to be deficient in any one of these micronutrients.

Even scarier is that if it's been a long time since you've taken high-quality vitamins or had an adequate intake of good nutrition daily, then according to Dr. Ames, your body is stealing your future life to keep you alive today. This is what is known as the Triage Theory.

The Triage Theory postulates that when adequate amounts of vitamins and minerals are limited, short-term survival takes precedence over functions whose loss can be better tolerated. In other words, your body will keep you alive today by breaking down and utilizing other parts of your body, such as your bones, muscle, skin, and other organs for the nutrients it needs now.

It is also established that if a person has a slow metabolism due to low nutrient levels, then the body's organs will also be functioning at a lower-than-optimal level. This means the entire body is then operating in survival mode due to a low-functioning metabolism, while experiencing a default of fat storage to conserve nutrient resources, and creeping closer to disease.

Dr. Ames also found that a deficiency of any of the critical micronutrients posed a threat of damage to the metabolism that was equal to, and in some circumstances greater than, the known damaging effects of radiation! (Sources: https://www.ncbi.nlm.nih.gov/pubmed/19692494, https://www.ncbi.nlm.nih.gov/pubmed/11295149)

Woah Nelly! Slow 'er down. Did that last statement impact you the way it did me? That being deficient in any of the essential micronutrients could have the same damage to my body as the known toxic effects of radiation? That's pretty serious stuff! This was enough for me to realize I needed to up my game in the nutrition department.

By the way, the signs of aging (sagging skin, deep wrinkles, fine lines, bags under the eyes, age spots, etc.) are just symptoms of a deficient metabolism. This is why you may see someone who is very unhealthy look about 20 years older than they actually are. This also explains why usually when you get healthier and lose weight, you inevitably end up looking much younger. Aging is simply a process that is determined by your metabolism. So not only will this program help you feel better and help you lose lots of inches, but it will also save you money on your beauty regimen. Who knew the answer to so many of our troubles lie in proper nutrition? Pretty cool.

To recap, there are 50 enzymes that do all the work of your metabolism and they need 40 essential micronutrients to function properly. What happens if you don't get these nutrients every day? Your metabolism slows down and goes into survival mode. When this happens, you start to age faster, get sick more often, and start gaining weight. This is also the beginning stage of disease.

As I've said multiple times throughout this book, fat is a symptom of a deeper underlying issue in the body and one of the major causes of fat storage is actually having a deficiency in certain nutrients. Even if you are already eating healthy foods and you are currently taking supplements, if you have weight to lose, it is a clear sign that you *aren't* eating the right foods and are not getting enough of the right nutrients.

I hope it is now crystal clear how important good nutrition is for your metabolism to be fast and efficient, allowing your body to come back into a state of balance and improve your overall health. The simplicity of it is that fat is created when the metabolism is not getting the nutrients it needs. Give your body what it needs, and the fat will no longer store and start to melt away!

This is what the 3X Program is all about. The whole basis of it is to nourish your body with everything it needs to bring your metabolism and your body back into complete balance.

We're now up to speed on our body's nutrient requirements, but how do you actually get those nutrients? Through good, high-quality nutrition *and* supplements.

The reason I highly recommend certain supplements is that our food supply (even when eating organic) is not what it used to be 50 years ago. The soil has been depleted and today's toxic environment and added stress to our body increases the nutritional requirements.

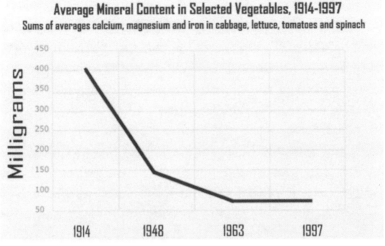

Average Mineral Content in Selected Vegetables, 1914-1997
Sums of averages calcium, magnesium and iron in cabbage, lettuce, tomatoes and spinach

Source: Lindlahr, 1914; Hamaker, 1982; U.S. Department of Agriculture, 1963 and 1997

A lot of people think they "get everything they need from what they eat." This is a general statement that drives me nuts. People who say this are speaking generally. Without knowing exactly what the quality of food is or with precisely how many nutrients it contains, there is no way to guarantee that a person gets everything they need from what they eat. It is utterly impossible to get therapeutic doses of nutrition (the amount you need to repair a metabolism) in a full day of meals, even if you are eating a perfect diet.

The National Health and Nutrition Examination Surveys (NHANES) has long reported that the food intake of the following groups of people in the United States does not provide adequate nutrition from all 40 essential nutrients for adequate health: the poor, teenagers, menstruating women, the obese, and the elderly. But they are now reporting, according to the Estimated Average Requirement (EAR), that micronutrient levels from food are probably not adequate for anyone else either, to express optimal health without disease.

"In my mind, there is no controversy. It is virtually impossible to get optimal nutrients for optimum health and aging from our diet. And you'll really be chronically deficient if you follow the RDA guidelines. Those were only designed to prevent illness, not to get you to your best health. If you follow them, you'll be deprived." – Al Sears, MD

There are multiple USDA studies that show that a substantial percentage of people are deficient in the essential micronutrients. Remember that these are the nutrients your metabolism needs to keep you healthy. We are not getting sufficient amounts of the nutrients we require from our food, so many people are deficient, and this is probably a large contributing factor to the fact that 70% of the population is either overweight or obese.

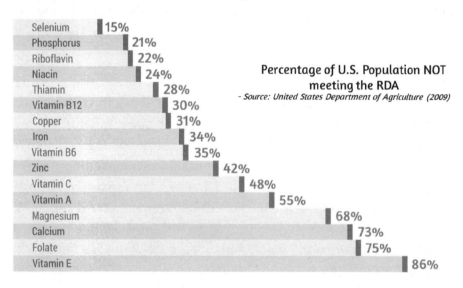

Percentage of U.S. Population NOT meeting the RDA
- *Source: United States Department of Agriculture (2009)*

In his book *Healthy for Life*, Dr. Ray Strand also notes that these nutrients are needed in greater amounts than can usually be obtained by food alone. In his practice, he has personally seen a reversal of Type 2 diabetes in hundreds of patients who optimize their nutrient intake with critical levels of vitamins, minerals, and essential fatty acids and who employ the lifestyle modifications described in his Healthy for Life program.

Thus far, you've learned that being overweight is a symptom of nutritional deficiencies that are causing your metabolism to slow down and store fat. As a result, a high-quality multi-vitamin is recommended as a low-cost preventative intervention in combination with the healthiest possible food choices. This is the best, low-cost option for optimal health and reducing the risk of common age-related diseases associated with obesity and ultimately death by secondary diseases of coronary heart disease and cancer. And not having enough micronutrients will signal to your body to start storing fat because it thinks it's starving.

This program is about getting your body into a long-lasting, healthy fat-burning mode because we want to fix the underlying issues of weight gain so that you can lose the weight and never gain it back.

To lose weight, it is very important that you not only start eating the right foods, but also support your metabolism with the nutrients it needs by taking good, high-quality supplements of all the essential vitamins and minerals your body needs.

The process begins with getting your body back in balance first. And THAT is the KEY and the "secret" to weight loss. With this information now under our belt, we'll delve deeper into the spectrum of factors that influence weight loss.

CHAPTER 4

OTHER FACTORS THAT INFLUENCE WEIGHT LOSS

HORMONES

As women, we have been made to believe that our hormones are evil and are just something that come to haunt us once a month, something we experience when we are pregnant, or when we're going through menopause. But our hormones are much, much more than that. Our hormones rule everything in our body and have for our entire life. I'm going to teach you the real truth about them and dispel common myths.

Simply put, hormones are nothing more than a communication sent from one part of your body to another. They are a critical component to weight loss because they control every system of your body, including the metabolism. They are also the primary reason why you either store fat or burn fat and can tell your metabolism to flip on your fat-burning or your fat-storing switch.

Also important to note is that calories don't control your metabolism; hormones do. Hormones such as insulin, cortisol, leptin, ghrelin, glucagon, estrogen, and thyroid to name a few are all responsible for your weight gain and your weight loss. It could be said that if your hormones are in balance, then you will be healthy and at a normal body weight. If your hormones are out of balance, you will experience less than optimal health and will most likely be overweight, or in some cases underweight. It is really that simple!

Here is how the hormone system works. It is basically just a communication system within the body. It is how your cells communicate to each other. Every one of your cells has hormone receptors on the outside of them, and each of those receptors receives hormones. As captured in the image below, the receptors are the circles on the outside of the cell.

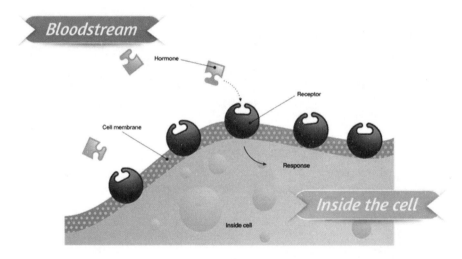

The hormone receptor's job is to receive communications (hormones) from certain glands in order to perform various functions that keep you alive and healthy.

Here's an example: A specific gland sends a communication to a specific cell. The cell receiving the hormone communication is called a "target" cell because the gland is actually targeting THAT one cell to receive its communication.

To help you better envision this process, think of it in terms of how a cell phone works. When you call a person, your phone is the gland and the person you are calling would be the target cell. As soon as you push the "call" or "send" button, that's the point that the gland secretes a hormone into the bloodstream. Your phone is the gland, the person's phone you're calling is the target cell, and what you say to the other person is the hormone. The hormone travels through the bloodstream to the target cell.

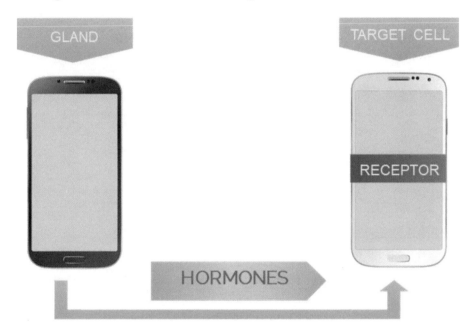

A gland can also receive a hormone message and a cell can send a hormone message. So full communication back and forth is possible. This is called a feedback loop.

Now, imagine what happens when you call someone's cell phone and they are in an area that doesn't have good cell reception. No connection is made, and you can't deliver your message to the person you're calling as intended.

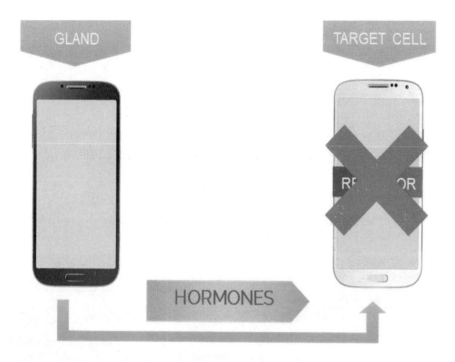

The same process can happen inside of your body when your hormone communication system isn't working properly.

Having bad cell reception is not a good thing given the fact that hormones regulate every aspect of our body and each receptor site has the power to alter our body's behavior in profound ways. These glands, hormones, and cell receptor sites *must* be in optimal shape and must be able to communicate to each other effectively if your body is going to be balanced.

WHAT IS A HORMONAL IMBALANCE?

The term "hormonal imbalance" means that your body is either producing too much or too little of certain hormones. It can also mean that your cells are not receiving your hormone communication.

Here are some of the most common signs and symptoms of hormone imbalances:

- Infertility and irregular periods
- Uncomfortable PMS symptoms (cramps, heavy bleeding, etc.)
- Unexplained weight gain or weight loss
- Depression and anxiety
- Fatigue
- Insomnia
- Low libido
- Digestive issues
- Hair loss and hair thinning

Symptoms of hormonal imbalances can range dramatically depending on what type of disorder or illness they cause. For example, hypothyroidism (or low thyroid) can cause a sluggish metabolism and contribute to problems like weight gain and low sex drive, whereas symptoms of adrenal fatigue often include anxiety and depression, trouble sleeping and fatigue.

Most hormonal imbalances are NOT genetic. They are actually heavily influenced by your lifestyle and your environment.

Here is a list of common triggers for hormone imbalance:

- ☐ Too much stress
- ☐ Not enough sleep
- ☐ The wrong types of exercise
- ☐ The wrong types of foods
- ☐ Toxins and endocrine disruptors

One of the great things about the 3X Program is that in it, we address all of these factors at the same time, bringing the hormones back into balance which allows maximum fat burning effects. This means you will not only lose a ton of weight, but you will be getting super healthy in the process.

THE #1 FAT STORING HORMONE

If there were just one thing I could tell you that would have the most impact on weight loss it would be to control the #1 top fat storing hormone, insulin.

Insulin is a fat storing hormone that is secreted by the pancreas. What triggers the pancreas to release insulin is glucose which is just a fancy name for sugar. Glucose comes from foods that are high in carbohydrates. The faster the carbohydrates get broken down into sugar the more insulin gets released.

Insulin's job is to take the glucose out of the bloodstream and store it into your cells. Your body can only store so much glucose in the cells before the rest has to be stored as fat.

Having too much glucose in your body at any given time is the #1 reason for fat storage because not only will insulin store glucose as fat but it also blocks your ability to burn fat.

I will discuss the effects of insulin and how to control it in an upcoming section but now it is important to know that this is one of the most crucial factors when it comes to being able to control your ability to lose weight effectively.

ENDOCRINE DISRUPTORS

Some of the most dangerous substances to your hormones are endocrine disruptors (endocrine is another word for hormone). An endocrine disruptor is something that your body confuses for a hormone because it has a similar molecular structure.

If you look at the image below you can see that the cell receptor sites accept the endocrine disruptor as if it were your hormone.

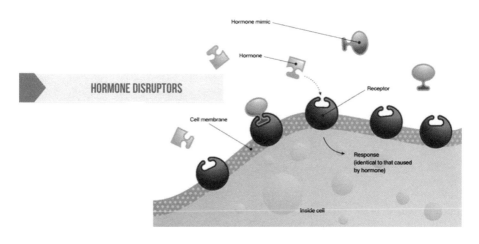

An example of an endocrine disruptor is soy. Soy has a molecular structure that is similar to the hormone estrogen. When you eat soy foods, your body actually thinks that it is estrogen, so it sets off a whole cascade of events when it receives the communication from it.

Any substance that the body thinks is estrogen (a fat-storing hormone) will react to it by throwing your reproductive hormones out of balance because of the excess estrogen coming through the system. This is known as estrogen dominance. Estrogen dominance is a hormone imbalance that can cause things like stubborn weight gain, migraines, PCOS, infertility, bad PMS symptoms (heavy bleeding, irregular cycles, and painful cramps) and can even lead to breast cancer.

Excess estrogen also blocks the thyroid from producing thyroid hormones and can cause an underactive thyroid. Here are some major endocrine disruptors that you will want to stay away from to avoid estrogen dominance.

☐ Pesticides, herbicides, insecticides (a major reason to consider eating organic food)

☐ Plastic bottled water (There are over 25,000 chemicals and hormone disruptors in plastic bottled water)

☐ Fluoride and chlorine which is in most city water supplies

☐ BPA from plastic water bottles, canned food, and other food packaging items (avoid processed foods)

☐ Soy in any form (soybean oil, soy milk, soy lecithin, etc.)

☐ Phlatates (found in plastics and fragrances)

☐ PEGs & parabens (found in most body care/skin care products)

You may not have realized this, but up until now, your own hormones have most likely been working against you, keeping you from being able to lose weight and having the body you want. It's not calories that you have to be concerned about, it's your hormone health. Having healthy hormones is *critical* to weight loss.

If you are feeling a bit overwhelmed by all of this information, don't worry. My point in telling you all this is so that you have a basic understanding of how your hormones and your metabolism effect your ability to lose weight. The good news is that if you follow this program, you will, by default, be doing all of the right things to support your metabolism and hormones to keep them healthy and balanced.

TOXINS

What is a toxin? I define it as any substance that has the potential to do damage to a living cell. Toxins in the form of chemical food flavoring enhancers, colors, preservatives, pesticides, growth hormones, and residues from countless prescription medicines in the city water supply have been shown to overwhelm the kidney and liver. They increase toxin overload and result in altered hormonal levels of insulin, glucagon, leptin, ghrelin, cortisol, and cortisone hormones that determine whether the body will store fat or release fat.

Excess weight is a combination of a nutritional deficiency, hormonal imbalances, and toxicity. There are not enough nutrients to keep the metabolism functioning optimally and too many toxins that interfere with normal hormone production. We will cover these in more depth, but for now, we'll delve deeper into the world of toxins.

Your body inherently knows what it needs to thrive, and Mother Nature provided us with food that contains the exact molecules that our body can recognize and use.

They're called "whole foods" and they come from the earth, plants, and animals, *not* from labs or manufacturing plants. Unfortunately, the majority of food that humans eat today isn't actually real food.

It is critical to understand that foods that don't fall into the categorization of whole foods are fake. And although they contain calories and can go in one end of your body and come out of the other, they do not have the essential nutrients that your body needs to survive optimally.

When you consume toxins or chemicals that are in the food you eat, your body can't ignore them and has to deal with them in one way or another. Doing so depletes your nutrient stores, thus toxins can create nutritional deficiencies. When your body is overburdened with toxins, it will begin to go into survival mode.

Because its priority is to survive, it will try to keep dangerous toxins away from your vital organs. It does this by manufacturing fat cells which get stored as the most dangerous type of fat, visceral fat. Visceral fat is body fat that is stored around a number of important internal organs such as the liver, pancreas, and intestines. To make it worse, your body thinks of burning fat as anti-survival, because it knows that burning fat will release these toxins back into your system. Equally important to know is that all excess weight contains a host of stored toxins. In fact, there are 1000 times more toxins stored in your fat cells than are in the rest of your body.

Toxins also severely alter the way your genes work and influence your hormones to a large degree, which also determine whether you will burn fat or store fat. This is why the first step of this program is detox. When I say detox, I am not referring to fasting for days on end or drinking a lemonade and cayenne pepper elixir. I am talking about eliminating toxins from your life before they even enter your body, which we do in the "remove foods" section of this program. The other aspect is through addressing the already-stored toxins in the digestive tract and fat cells, which we do over a period of time with good nutrition, adequate hydration, and supplementation.

With a better understanding of toxins under your belt, we're going to go over some of the most common food toxins so that you are aware of how they affect your health. This information will aid you in making better-informed decisions for yourself in the future.

If you ate something poisonous like cyanide, you would die immediately, and it would have been pretty obvious what had caused you to die. Well, what happens when you eat food that contains smaller amounts of poisons? You might not die instantly when you eat, but that doesn't mean that the poisons in those small amounts aren't accumulating over time and causing a lot of problems that could eventually end up causing the same outcome, only slower.

The exposure to and buildup of food toxins within our bodies most certainly contributes to weight gain, accelerated aging, and declining health. The gradual detrimental effects as a result of toxins are often overlooked because we have a tendency to expect results immediately, but those are what we have to pay the most attention to!

THE STATE OF TODAY'S FOOD

The majority of today's processed food is created intentionally to get you to eat more of it. There is very little consideration put into how it will fuel your body to be strong, work optimally, grow, and survive. The more you eat, the more you buy, and the more profit the food company amasses. The bottom line in their strategy is ensuring that the taste is addictive enough to keep you coming back, not your health. And commercials with lines like, "Betcha can't eat just one," and, "Once you pop, you can't stop," make clear what their focus is.

Food manufacturers achieve this goal of getting you addicted to the unhealthy stuff by creating food with addictive chemicals like flavor enhancers, artificial colorings, preservatives, and even fragrances. Yes, it's a whole process! What's worse is that **these chemicals placed into our food have never been tested for human safety and they are not regulated** whatsoever. It's no surprise that many of the thousands of chemicals that are placed into our food have been shown to cause obesity and other metabolic diseases in field studies.

You're probably wondering how food manufacturers get away with this. If it were so bad for us, it couldn't be sold on the grocery store shelf right? *Wrong.* Believe it or not, the food in America is not regulated the way we trust that it is. Many other countries have banned a lot of the chemicals that we allow in our food. As consumers, we really have no idea what is going into our food and we eat it blindly, all the while believing it is "safe."

Michael Taylor, the FDA's deputy commissioner for food safety, has said "We simply do not have the information to vouch for the safety of many of these chemicals. We do not know the volume of particular chemicals that are going into the food supply." *He* is from the FDA—our governing body for food and drugs, the source that is supposed to be the most reliable—and he is basically admitting that there are no regulations on what goes into our food.

Another important point of consideration is that we have deceptive labeling on our foods. Did you know that food manufacturers can put anything they want on the packaging? It's true! They can call it healthy, natural, lite, sugar-free, fat-free, or whatever the new buzzword of the moment is. You can be certain that manufacturers will include it on their package to entice you into buying it.

If you ever looked at the ingredients on the back of the foods you often eat, you will find a long list of things that you couldn't pronounce if your life depended on it. Most people do not know what half of these ingredients actually are or what to look for to know whether something is dangerous to their health or not. And sadly, even when we do know what to look out for and avoid, we are still misled by labeling loopholes and the fact that some ingredients aren't even required to be labeled. For example, the front of the package might say, "healthy," but the list of ingredients (or what's not listed) is anything but healthy.

WHAT'S REALLY IN OUR FOOD?

That said, it really makes you question what you're ingesting, right? I mean, here we are trying our best to be healthy and we have no idea what is actually in the food that we are eating! Unfortunately, the bad news doesn't stop there. Trans fats, which we hear a lot about these days, are an example of ingredients that are toxic yet are in many foods we eat that are labeled as "healthy," or "diet-friendly." Before we continue on the topic of trans fats, it is important to note that they are not the same as saturated fats. For a long time, these two types of fats have been incorrectly lumped together as bad fats.

Saturated fats that come from coconut oil and animal fat are natural fats that are solid at room temperature and contain small amounts of trans fats but these are not the type of trans fats that are bad for you. Man-made trans fats, on the other hand, come from highly processed liquid vegetable oils that have been chemically altered by adding hydrogen to them, which make them solid at room temperature. The high processing and forcing of hydrogen into the fat molecules alter them in a way that is very damaging to the body. Have you noticed the trend of how damaging man-made foods are to our bodies?

Trans fats are toxic to the cell membranes, causing the cells to become leaky and distorted. This can promote vitamin and mineral deficiencies, among many other problems. Furthermore, trans fats have been linked to weight gain.

"Diets rich in trans fats cause a redistribution of fat tissue into the abdomen and lead to a higher body weight, even when the total dietary calories are controlled," said Lawrence L. Rudel, Ph.D.

Additionally, consuming partially hydrogenated vegetable oils and the trans fats that are formed with this process has been linked to increases in cancer, heart disease, and many other chronic degenerative disorders.

Because the general public has caught on to the fact that trans fats are bad for us, the FDA made it a requirement for food manufacturers to label any food product as having trans fat in it. They stipulate that you have to label your product as having trans fats in it *only* if you have a certain amount of trans fat per serving. In order to circumvent these regulations, because obviously, the food manufacturer doesn't want to label their product as unhealthy (though it is), they lower the serving size so they do not have to claim there are any trans fats in their product. Tricky, right? You would be sickened if you knew the amount of food that is currently on the grocery store shelves that have trans fats in them but are not labeled as such. However, the food manufacturers do not want to label trans fats because then we wouldn't purchase their food.

The next time you go grocery shopping, I want you to be aware of the most common foods made with trans fats:

- Peanut butter
- Pre-made cookies and desserts
- Donuts
- Margarine
- Cake icing (any anything else creamy or spreadable)
- Fried food is most likely made with trans fats

Take a look at this example of a label from a very popular peanut butter brand:

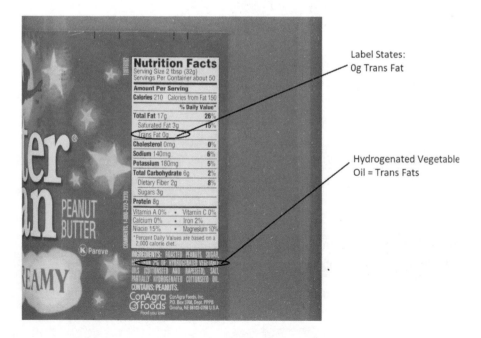

To the untrained eye, a person may think, "Hey this is just healthy ole peanut butter, made straight from peanuts." But what they don't realize is that the ingredient "hydrogenated vegetable oils" contains trans fats!

MORE HIDDEN TOXIC INGREDIENTS

Another example of something toxic that you will find in many foods is deceptively labeled MSG. MSG stands for Monosodium Glutamate and is also known as "hydrolyzed protein" (*hydro* from "hydrogen" and *lyzed*, which means "breaking down" or "breaking down protein by use of hydrogen").

MSG is a food additive that was invented by Japanese scientists back in 1908 when they discovered that the seaweed they had been using to flavor their food for hundreds of years had an active ingredient called "glutamic acid." They decided to create synthetic glutamic acid so that they could add it to all their foods to enhance the flavor, instead of using the natural form of glutamic acid found in seaweed.

The scientists achieved this by taking a protein from vegetables (seaweed), meat, beef, chicken, or soy and breaking it down chemically into its amino-acid parts. Once they break down the protein into amino acids, glutamic acid is produced, which, depending on which protein was broken down, produces a certain type of flavoring.

Food manufacturers went bananas when this was discovered because they saw a financial opportunity where they could create fake, processed foods and use MSG to make them taste real. MSG also has addictive properties and would cause people to want to continue to eat their food. Dr. Mercola of www.drmercola.com says it's a silent killer that's worse than alcohol, nicotine, and drugs. Dr. Russell Blaylock, a board-certified neurosurgeon, describes MSG as a dangerous excitotoxin, which means that it overexcites your cells to the point of damage, acting as a poison. Sadly, even infant formulas and baby food contain this poison, despite the fact that babies and infants are four times more sensitive than adults to the toxic effects of this chemical.

You now know that toxins are bad for you and act as a poison, but it's equally as important to know how the toxins from consuming MSG can manifest. Eating foods containing MSG can signal to your body to produce visceral fat, the most dangerous type that surrounds your organs. It can also increase your risk of heart attack, stroke, insomnia, Type 2 diabetes, and more.

According to Dr. Berg, author of "The New Body Type Guide", in animal studies, MSG has been shown to increase insulin output by 300%. Again, insulin is a fat-storing hormone that not only makes additional fat on your body but prevents fat burning from occurring.

MSG is also a probable contributor to the growing obesity epidemic. As the FDA continues to vouch for its safety, scientists have known that MSG causes obesity since the 1960s! A study was conducted that showed that women who ate MSG were three times more overweight than those who didn't. You can read the full study for yourself at http://sph.unc.edu/unc-researchers-find-msg-use-linked-to-obesity/.

A shocking 95% of processed foods contain MSG! The confusing part is that MSG is not usually labeled as "MSG." You will find it under the name of Monosodium Glutamate, Hydrolyzed Protein, or any of the other 40 different names that it can be noted as. MSG is hidden in food labels under such things as broth, casein, hydrolyzed, autolyzed, and more, making it extremely difficult to identify. A good rule of thumb to follow on how to identify this toxin is that chances are if it's a processed food in a package, it contains MSG.

Here is a list of the most common types of food that contain MSG:

- Packaged snack items (chips, crackers, flavored nuts, peanuts)
- Bouillon cubes, sauce mixes, condiments, salad dressings, , BBQ sauce, etc.
- Most processed convenience foods (TV dinners, dehydrated soup mixes, rice mixes, tofu)
- Many processed meat products
- Almost all canned soups

The bottom line is that no one is really looking out for your best interest when it comes to what is being put into your food. Therefore, the only person who you can trust to know what's in your food is you. Learning to read food labels is a skill that I would recommend making a priority of immediately. Otherwise, you will be making uniformed choices and will be accidentally poisoning yourself and your family with these food toxins. This acquired skill will enable and empower you to make the healthiest purchasing decisions when it comes to choosing foods that will help you get healthy and lose weight.

I couldn't possibly cover all of the 10,000 chemicals that are in the ingredients of the foods sold in the grocery store, so the good news is that just by removing the foods that I recommend in the next chapter, you will be eliminating all of them by default! Before we move to that section though, I do want to talk about one more, and probably the worst, labeling "loophole" in this chapter: GMOs.

GENETICALLY MODIFIED ORGANISMS

We hear a lot about genetically modified organisms (GMO), but what exactly are they? A GMO is the result of a laboratory process where genes from the DNA of one species are extracted and artificially forced into the genes of an unrelated plant or animal. The foreign genes may come from bacteria, viruses, insects, animals, or even humans.

It is most used in the agricultural industry to make a crop to be pesticide and herbicide resistant. Genetically modified organisms are all engineered as "Roundup-ready crops." Roundup is a brand of herbicide/pesticide and it's a very popular weed killer. Farmers purchase these Round-up ready seeds from a company called Monsanto—the same manufacturer as Roundup. This allows a large amount of weed killer and pesticides to be sprayed on a crop and because the crop has been genetically modified, it will only kill the weeds and pests, not the crop. There is then less crop failure, more crops to sell, and more cost savings for Monsanto.

ARE GMOS SAFE?

The active ingredient in Roundup is a chemical called glyphosate. Glyphosate was originally used as a descaling agent by Stanford Chemicals in the 1960s, which used it to get all of the mineral sediments out of industrial pipes and boilers. When they went to dispose of the glyphosate in nature, they found that whatever it touched was completely annihilated. All the plants, weeds, and any living organism it touched died.

Let me explain exactly how all of this works. Remember earlier when I was talking about our metabolism relying on enzymes? Well, all organisms, including plants, humans, and animals, depend on enzymes to process protein that is necessary for survival. Those enzymes do specific things that keep us alive and one of the things they do is process the protein that we take in. It is one of the many metabolic processes that keep us alive, but for plants and smaller organisms, it's one of only a few processes that keep them alive.

There is a metal in the center of the molecule of this necessary enzyme. The way glyphosate works is that it binds to the metal that is in the center of the enzyme and it makes that enzyme unable to synthesize or process protein. The organism then dies, because it needs the protein for its survival and can't live without these enzymes doing the job of synthesizing protein.

When it was developed and approved for consumption, there was an erroneous belief that the enzyme it inhibits in plants is not found in animals or humans; that is untrue. Absorption of nutrients in animals and humans is via the gut microbiome (the collective genome of organisms inhabiting our body), which has the identical enzyme system as plants. This means that glyphosate has the same effect on the good bacteria in our gut responsible for digestion and absorption of nutrients as it does on plants. This equals total destruction. The World Health Organization (WHO) recently classified glyphosate as a "probable human carcinogen." You can find more on this at:

http://www.academia.edu/6495617/Glyphosate_is_an_antibiotic_and_Japanese_knotweed_is_a_Glyphosate-Resistant_GR_Superweed.

The effects of glyphosate create a widespread problem, as studies have shown that even at extremely low amounts, it can cause breast cancer. This includes what the government calls "safe" limits of glyphosate that are allowed to be in our food and drinking water. If you visit www.feedtheworld.info you can read a study in which 0.1 parts of glyphosate per billion parts of water produced an increase of mammary tumors and alterations of liver and kidneys in mice. Despite these facts, the US government allows 700 parts of glyphosate per billion parts of our drinking water, which is 7000 times the amount that has been shown to increase breast cancer.

Several popular cereal brands were recently tested for glyphosate levels and the levels were off the charts at 1,125.3

parts per billion! That is almost double the amount allowed in our drinking water and 10,000 times the amount that increases breast cancer.

Studies completed in 2014 showed that glyphosate is found in American women's breastmilk and urine. But due to the testing method used in these tests, the Environmental Protection Agency (EPA and other government regulators simply ignored the results as if they weren't substantial evidence.

It gets worse. Glyphosate was registered as an antibiotic in 2010. We all know that antibiotics are usually prescribed when we need to get rid of a bad bacterial infection. However, antibiotics do not just selectively kill the bad bacteria; they also destroy the good bacteria that we need to keep us healthy. Did you know that 80% of our immune system is in our digestive tract and it is the microorganisms, or good bacteria, in our gut that determine how often we get sick?

They are what fight off bad bacteria, pathogens, viruses, and parasites. If we are continually exposed to antibiotics, then we kill off the very things we need to keep us alive, functioning, and healthy. And good bacteria do more than fight off diseases; they digest our food, help us absorb nutrients, and even affect our mood. By eating GMOs and food that is sprayed with glyphosate, you will essentially be exposing yourself to harmful antibiotics on a continual basis.

Since GMOs have entered our food supply, there has been an almost direct correlation between GMOs and the increase in hypertension (high blood pressure), obesity, diabetes, neurological disorders (autism, Alzheimer's, Parkinsons, senile dementia), auto-immune disorders (Hashimotos's, rheumatoid arthritis, etc., inflammatory bowel diseases (ulcerative colitis, Crohn's disease, Irritable Bowel Syndrome, and certain cancers like thyroid and liver cancer.

All of the correlations were greater than 90%, with autism and senile dementia at 99%, an almost exact correlation between the two datasets. For further information, visit this website: http://gmofreewashington.com/our-experts/nancy-swanson/.

WHAT CAN YOU DO ABOUT IT?

When I first heard about GMOs five years ago, I didn't really think they were a big deal because I truly believed that the government was looking out for our best interests and never believed that something so horrifying would be allowed to be put in our food. I felt overwhelmed with all of this new information and I was also mad that this has happened to our food.

I felt scared and a little bit betrayed, to be honest. I almost wished I hadn't learned about all this because it seemed easier to just not believe it or not know about it. As they say, ignorance is bliss, right? Well, ignorance is only bliss until reality smacks you in the face and makes you wake up. The truth is, knowledge is power and it's only after you are educated about something that you can do anything about it.

I do not like to live my life in fear and feel that there is nothing I can do about a certain situation. I'm always trying to find ways to take responsibility for my life and figure out what I can do to make life better with what I can control. So I embarked on a journey to better educate myself. It took me years of doing research and watching various videos and documentaries that were showing the real science behind GMOs and what they are doing to our health for me to finally realize that this isn't just a conspiracy theory.

The more research I did, the more I learned that the single best thing I could do for my health is to make sure the food I was eating was not genetically modified. I also realized that I *can* control the food that I put into my mouth and the food I feed my family; I do make that choice. It might not be easy to do all the time, but it would be a heck of a lot easier to try the best I can than to deal with getting sick or being overweight for my entire life not realizing why.

I came to the conclusion that when grocery shopping I would buy all organic food because, in the US, there is really only one way to know whether or not you are eating GMOs: If you do not eat organic, you are consuming GMOs. If you eat organic food, it is not allowed to be genetically modified or sprayed with glyphosate. I also did not want to support manufacturers that were deliberately putting toxic chemicals into our food by giving my money to them when I buy food. Supply and demand, right?

The more people who buy toxic food, the cheaper it will be. The more people who buy organic and support the local farmers who are producing food the way it was meant to be made, the cheaper it will eventually be.

Due to the prevalence of GMOs in our food supply, I knew that it was unrealistic that I would never come into contact with them and I didn't want to spend my life being stressed out all the time about what is in my food. There is a healthy median between enjoying your life while doing the best you can to stay as healthy as possible. So here is what I do to maintain that balance.

- I avoid all processed foods. 85% of processed foods are made with GMO ingredients. That alone is the single biggest thing you can do to avoid GMOs.

- When I grocery shop, I buy 100% organic food or local food that even though isn't certified organic, was still produced in the same manner as organic food. (In the last section of this book I will show you incredible ways to eat organic without spending any more money than you currently are on your groceries.)
- I avoid all bread (all wheat is doused in glyphosate right before harvest)
- I do not drink soda (high fructose corn syrup is made from GMOs)
- I make sure that I don't randomly snack on chips or other snacks out of boredom. If I am hungry I eat a meal made up of protein and vegetables and stay away from putting unnecessary food items into my body.
- When I eat out or travel, I just make the best choices I can since there is no way I can completely avoid them.

If you follow this program and avoid all of the foods that I am going to discuss next, you will, by default, be avoiding a lot of GMOs so you really won't have to actively think about it.

Here are some additional things you can do about GMOs:

1. Eat at home as much as possible. Make food at home from sources that you trust.

2. Eat foods high in probiotics to help replenish your gut from any damage that is done from the antibiotic properties of glyphosate.

3. Get educated and educate others. That is the only way that the situation of having a toxic food supply in the US and around the world is going to change.

4. Support groups and organizations that are trying to make a difference. Shop at local health food stores or seek out the local farmers. Go to the Farmer's Market. Start supporting the people who are doing things right versus continuing to support these big corporations who have proven to us clearly, over and over again, that it is not us that they care about.

SECTION 2

THE 3X WEIGHT LOSS PLAN

CHAPTER 5

GET HEALTHY TO LOSE WEIGHT

I've covered a lot thus far, but everything can be summarized by one statement: *You need to get healthy before you can lose real weight and keep it off for good.* Most people erroneously believe the opposite of that though, which is that they need to lose weight (first) in order to be healthy. So they focus all their efforts on weight loss and do various diets and exercise programs, yet are confused when results don't follow. Again, once you fix the broken balancing mechanism within the metabolism, weight loss will occur naturally as a result of having a healthier body. The first step toward a healthier lifestyle and balanced body is to remove fat-storing foods.

REMOVING FAT-STORING FOODS

What is a fat-storing food? A fat-storing food is any food that will cause your body to store fat. A fat-storing food is one that can also stop your body from burning fat. Most people believe that eating too many calories or eating fat is what caused them to be fat, but this is not true. It is certain foods that cause you to store fat and certain foods that will allow you to burn fat. It is not based on the number of calories in those foods, but rather the hormonal response and chemical reaction those foods produce once inside your body.

For the fat-burning phase of this program and to get the best results, you will want to completely remove all fat-storing foods.

There are a lot of diet programs that tell you to eat certain foods and to not eat other foods with no explanation why. This makes dieting so confusing because every diet has different views on what is healthy or not. But remember, you don't have to worry about deciphering anything. The 3X Program is as simple and straightforward as it gets, and throughout this book, I will take the guesswork out of these concepts.

Every food you put into your mouth (whether it is considered healthy or not either triggers your body to store fat or burn fat. You could be eating all of the right healthy foods, but if you include any wrong foods you will simply not lose weight. This section is very important because it could mean the difference between burning fat and getting amazing results or storing fat and not losing the weight that you want. Remember, food is information and that information instructs the body to do something. It will tell the body to either store fat or it will tell it body to burn fat.

This can be tricky to figure out on your own because foods that may be considered "healthy" can actually keep you from being able to burn fat. To get the best results from your efforts, it is key to know which foods to eat and which ones to stay away from.

"Everything in moderation" simply does not work when it comes to weight loss. I had to learn this the hard way. This was the problem I had when I was trying to lose weight. I didn't understand why I wasn't getting results when I was eating so healthy and exercising all the time. I thought that if I ate really healthy and worked out every day that I deserved to eat whatever I wanted on the weekends. I later learned that it wasn't about calories and that by doing certain things I was throwing my body *out* of fat-burning mode and making it impossible to lose weight, no matter how hard I was trying. Once you have reached your goal and have the body you want, then yes, moderation is possible. But not until you get to that point, otherwise you will not see results and will be spinning your wheels and will spend the rest of your life trying to get there.

Some of the following fat-storing foods that I recommend eliminating are included because they cause addictions and cravings, which makes it hard to stick to eating in a healthy way. Since one of your goals is to get rid of the cravings and the bad addictions to these foods, we will be removing those as well. And then of course, as mentioned in the last section, there are certain foods that contain toxins or ingredients that have a negative impact on your digestive system, hormones, and metabolism (all of which control your weight loss).

Below is a list of foods that I highly recommend avoiding during the rapid fat loss phase. Now when you first see this list of foods, don't think, "Oh no! I can't do this. All of these foods are staples in my household. There is no way I can get rid of all of these!" Please be rest assured that you *can* get rid of these foods and still cook for yourself and your family or still go out to eat and still enjoy your life! I promise. Nowadays there are so many recipes and healthier alternatives to use in place of unhealthy foods. At the end of this chapter, I have provided you with a "substitution list" of bad foods to swap out for healthier versions. So don't worry, this program is totally doable. Just keep going and read until the end and you will see! Some of these foods (such as dairy, alcohol, and some grains) can be re-introduced once you are at your ideal body weight, but my advice would be to mostly eliminate the rest of these items from your life if you want to maintain your results and have great health.

Foods to remove:
- ☐ All processed foods
- ☐ Diet foods

- ☐ Grains and gluten products
- ☐ Sugar and artificial sweeteners
- ☐ Processed vegetable oils
- ☐ Soy products
- ☐ Dairy products
- ☐ Alcohol

PROCESSED FOODS AND DIET FOODS

In talking about the foods listed above, you'll notice that I mentioned that they should be consumed as infrequently as possible. Processed foods, however, are a completely different story. These need to go immediately and **forever!**

Processed foods are packaged foods that have a ton of bad ingredients that can destroy your health and keep you from losing weight. This is because they are completely dead food. There is absolutely nothing in processed foods that your body can actually use. There are only empty calories that trick you into thinking you are full, but then trigger cravings that come back with a vengeance.

Sadly, 90% of what you find on the grocery store shelves are man-made foods that are mostly harmful, addictive, and making you fat. Chips, crackers, pretzels, cereals, cookies, bottled condiments, frozen meals, and more all fall into this category.

Processed foods are addicting because they stimulate the pleasure centers in the brain, so we overeat them. This is because they are engineered to be rewarding to the brain and bring us pleasure, versus natural whole foods that are intended for sustenance. Once we are hooked on these foods as a result of their hyper-rewarding nature, we crave them, need them, and our appetites gravitate towards them.

3X WEIGHT LOSS   Laura Sales

This aspect of addiction is something that should be taken very seriously. Because of the aforementioned reasons in this and the last chapter, we understand that eating these non-whole foods habitually is a very slippery slope. Food addiction is a very serious condition that, if not curbed, controlled, and dealt with, can have horrendous effects on people's health and life.

These addictions always revolve around junk food, sweets, and unhealthy fatty and salty foods because they activate pleasure and reward centers in the brain just like heroin and cocaine. Notice how no one becomes addicted to spinach and how you usually won't find yourself binge eating on wild salmon or vegetables?

Processed foods, because of their highly addictive nature, will likely be hard to give up in the beginning. You may even experience withdrawal symptoms such as fatigue and headaches. This is all normal and will only last a few days though. If you eat the foods I recommend and use the supplements I suggest, you will experience fewer symptoms and get through the detox period a lot easier. And once you have these toxic processed foods out of your life for good, you will experience a myriad of health benefits and won't believe how fast the fat melts off of your body!

The effects of these foods on your body cause such a heavy burden because they are not real foods and thus are hard to break down. They damage your gut, slow your metabolism, and throw your hormones out of whack. They are made with GMOs and loaded with MSG, soy, sugar, high fructose corn syrup, artificial sweeteners, trans fats, and other harmful ingredients.

Nature never intended us to consume processed foods and if you look at the statistics from the introduction of processed foods into the food supply and the increase in obesity in the population, they almost completely correlate. **So the single most important thing you can do for your health and to lose weight and keep**

it off for good is to quit eating processed foods. This is also the quickest way to lose weight and this one step alone will completely change your health and your body!

Diet food is also a processed food, but it's marketed to us as being healthy or diet-friendly. Things like margarine, low-fat yogurt, diet soda, artificial sweeteners, protein bars, energy drinks, vitamin waters, and fat-free salad dressings are labeled to make us think that they're going to assist us in losing weight. But it's not what is labeled on the front of the package that matters. Remember, food manufacturers can put anything they want on the front of their package. What matters is the list of ingredients on the back of the package.

GRAIN AND GLUTEN PRODUCTS

Our purpose in this phase is to remove all foods that will stop or slow weight loss. So the next food to eliminate during the fat-burning phase are all grains such as flour, bread, pasta, wheat, rice, oats, corn, etc. Why? Because grains contain very high amounts of fat-storing carbohydrates and so they halt weight loss. This is true whether the grain is a simple or complex carbohydrate.

In fact, eating a piece of whole wheat bread (complex carbohydrate) has a worse effect on blood sugar levels than eating a Snickers bar (simple carbohydrate). The difference between a simple carb and a complex carb is only the amount of time it takes to digest. But regardless of the type of carb, once the body breaks it down into glucose it is nothing but sugar.

I know many women who mistakenly think they are being health conscious by having a turkey sandwich on whole wheat bread. They have been told that complex carbohydrates are good for them and that eating whole grains are a healthy choice when trying to lose weight. This is one of the biggest dieting mistakes. Here is what *really* happens when you eat these types of "healthy" food.

When consuming foods that contain high amounts of carbohydrates (regardless if it is complex or simple), once digested they turn to glucose (sugar) and enter your bloodstream. Once in your bloodstream, your pancreas senses the rise in glucose and releases the fat-storage hormone insulin to get rid of it. Insulin's job is to take the glucose (sugar) from your bloodstream and store it into your muscle cells and liver cells and whatever is left over gets stored as fat. It literally creates fat cells to have a place to store the glucose. The catch is that the only way glucose can go into muscle cells or the liver cells is if there is room for it!

With the average person eating the standard American diet, most of the time there is no room in their cells for glucose. This is because every cell is already stuffed full of glucose from the previous meal. Because of the high-carbohydrate meal they had for breakfast (oatmeal, muffins, yogurt, orange juice, toast, bagels, fruit, etc.), lunch (bread, tortilla wraps, etc.), and dinner (potatoes, rice, pasta, etc.), every cell is already packed with glucose and so everything they eat gets stored as fat. This is the basic flows of how fat storage occurs.

For you to lose fat effectively you need to convert your body from a sugar-burning metabolism (which means constantly burning glucose from the last meal you had) over to a fat-burning metabolism (where the body has to use fat cells for energy). The way to do this is to remove certain fat-causing carbohydrates. Otherwise, your body will never have a chance to tap into your stored fat and use it as energy.

Now notice I said *certain carbs* and *not all carbs*. It is true that your body needs carbs, the brain simply cannot function without them. When we get into the fat-burning foods section of this book, you will learn about the healthy carbs you can have that will help you lose weight.

Most people who are overweight have several hormonal imbalances going on and removing certain carbohydrates greatly reduces the stress on these hormones, allowing for a more balanced situation so that fat burning can occur.

Removing all carbs or choosing the wrong ones can completely sabotage your hormones and your weight-loss results. A no-carb diet can result in shutting down of the thyroid, muscle loss, no fat loss, not feeling satisfied after meals, cravings, and digestive problems. This is why I do not recommend a completely no-carb diet.

On the other hand, eating too many of the wrong carbs also causes hormonal imbalances, fat storage, excess hunger, cravings, and energy crashes throughout the day, all which lead to an increase in weight gain. In fact, most people eat twice as many carbohydrates than they are able to use, a big reason why 70% of Americans are either overweight or obese. This is why it is critical to find the right balance of the right carbs. You will learn which carbs I recommend in the fat-burning foods section.

SUGAR & ARTIFICIAL SWEETENERS

Speaking of carbohydrates, the next food to remove is sugar. This includes not only white processed sugar, but also sugar alternatives like honey, agave, coconut sugar, maple syrup, molasses, cane sugar, and high-sugared fruits (a list of approved fruits will be provided). Even though fruit is healthy and contains a lot of vitamins and minerals, if you want to lose weight, you should not eat them. Fruit is loaded with sugar and if there is any sugar in your body, it will immediately shut down any and all fat-burning hormones and will cause you to store fat.

Aside from sugar most definitely causing weight gain, it also makes you age a lot faster and look older than you really are. This is the result of AGEs (advanced glycation end products). This happens when a chemical reaction causes sugar to interfere with the protein in the body, resulting in damage to healthy tissues, causing them to age quicker. Eating sugar also causes your body to break down collagen and elastin in your skin, which results in wrinkly, sagging skin.

All artificial sweeteners like aspartame and sucralose are a big no-no because research has shown that consuming artificial sweeteners causes a cascade of negative effects to your metabolism. Research published in *PLOS One* found that regularly consuming artificially sweetened soft drinks is associated with several disorders of metabolic syndrome, including:

- ☐ Abdominal obesity
- ☐ Insulin resistance
- ☐ Impaired glucose intolerance
- ☐ Abnormally elevated fats in the blood
- ☐ High blood pressure

The study found that drinking aspartame-sweetened diet soda daily increased the risk of Type 2 diabetes by 67% (regardless of whether they gained weight or not) and the risk of metabolic syndrome by 36%.

Research published in *Applied Physiology, Nutrition, and Metabolism* found that aspartame intake is associated with greater glucose intolerance in people with obesity. Glucose intolerance is a where your body loses its ability to deal with high amounts of sugar and is a well-known precursor to Type 2 diabetes. It also plays a role in obesity, because the excess sugar in your blood ends up being stored in your fat cells.

This means that obese individuals who use aspartame may have higher blood sugar levels, which in turn will raise insulin levels, leading to related weight gain, inflammation, and an increased risk of diabetes. So please avoid all artificial sweeteners.

You may use natural, sugar-free sweeteners like plant-based stevia, monk fruit, erythritol and xylitol.

DAIRY

Next food to remove is dairy, including low-fat and non-fat milk, yogurt, and cheese. The main reason to remove dairy is because most dairy contains growth hormones that were given to the cows. These growth hormones are used to fatten them up to get them to produce more milk. If you eat dairy that came from a cow that had growth hormones, chances are that it will fatten you up, too.

Aside from that, dairy is also an acidic food that slows down digestion and causes bloating. It interferes with the removal of toxins and can cause inflammation which blocks your ability to burn fat.

PROCESSED VEGETABLE OILS

There are a lot of clever marketing strategies that lead us to believe that cheaply produced vegetable oils such as canola oil, soybean oil, and corn oil are better for us than the eating real fats like lard, butter, coconut oil, etc. but unfortunately, they are anything but.

One of the major problems with vegetable oils is that they are extremely high in omega-6 linolenic acids and do not have a sufficient amount of omega-3's. And research has recently shown that having an imbalance or incorrect ratio of omega-6 to omega-3 can result in increased tendency to form blood clots, inflammation, high blood pressure, irritation of the digestive tract, depressed immune function, sterility, cell proliferation, cancer, and weight gain.

Despite the name "vegetable oil," these oils do not come from vegetables. They actually come from genetically modified seeds and are *highly* processed. In the refining process, these vegetable oils go rancid. With their murky gray color and rancid smell they are not very appealing to the end consumer, and so they are bleached, deodorized, and clarified using high levels of heat and toxic chemicals which cause inflammation and oxidative stress (free radicals). The end product is a rancid, highly toxic bad fat that is bad for your brain, body, and ultimately dangerous to your health. All of this is despite the heart-healthy claims.

Unfortunately, a lot of foods today have vegetable oils hidden in them. And all processed foods will contain one or more of these bad fats along with trans fats, which are the worst kind. Most restaurants cook their food in vegetable oil and 99% of salad dressings contain canola or soybean oil. "Salad oil," by the way, is nothing but a mixture of canola and soybean oil, so don't be fooled!

Please avoid the following vegetable oils:

- Corn oil
- Cottonseed oil
- Soybean oil
- Canola oil
- Margarine
- Anything oil that contains trans fats

SOY PRODUCTS

The next food to get rid of is soy (soy milk, soy cheese, soy meat-substitute, tofu, soybeans, soybean oil, soy lecithin, etc.) Soy is promoted as being a healthier alternative to meat and dairy and as beneficial to weight loss, but it's actually neither healthy nor beneficial to weight loss.

Soy is an endocrine disruptor because the body confuses soy for the hormone estrogen, and in this way, throws your natural hormones out of balance. Estrogen is a fat-storing hormone and most of us have way too much estrogen (known as estrogen dominance) due to exposure to toxins, pesticides and things like BPA, which is in all plastic and canned foods. Soy also blocks the thyroid gland from producing thyroid hormones.

ALCOHOL

Alcohol contributes heavily to weight gain because when there's alcohol present, your body burns the alcohol instead of fat. The effect is very similar to how sugar is acknowledged and processed in your body. If there's alcohol in your body, it is going to shut off your fat-burning ability.

The consumption of alcohol also causes an increase in the hormone cortisol. Cortisol is a fat-storing hormone, which causes you to gain fat around the midsection.

One last point about alcohol is that it is damaging to the liver, which is already most likely suffering due to being overweight and having excess toxins. The liver is responsible for over five hundred different functions, including the conversion of foods and supporting the fat-burning hormones. The best things you can do for your liver is to nourish it with high-quality nutrition and eliminate as many toxins as possible.

FOOD SUBSTITUTION LISTS

Here is a short list of foods that you can substitute for healthier versions:

INSTEAD OF THIS:	HAVE THIS:
Diet Soda	Zevia Soda or Flavored Carbonated Water
Margarine or grain fed butter	Grass Fed Ghee (Clarified butter)
Protein Bars	Grass Fed Beef Jerky (no sugar added)
Regular Mayonnaise	Avocado Oil Mayonnaise—Primal Kitchen
Corn or Flour Tortillas	Almond Flour or Coconut Flour Tortillas
Potato Chips	Homemade Kale Chips (or other vegetable)
Oatmeal	Make a "granola" with crushed nuts and chia seeds
Crackers	Almond Flour or Flax Seed Crackers
Rice	Cauliflower Rice or Quinoa
White Flour	Coconut Flour, Almond Flour or Cassava Flour
Wheat Noodles	Spaghetti Squash or Spiralized Vegetable Noodles
White Potatoes	Sweet Potatoes or Steamed Cauliflower
Dairy Milk	Almond Milk (or other nut milk)
Cheese	Cashew Cheese or Nutritional Yeast
Yogurt	Coconut Milk Yogurt or Coconut Kefir
Fruit Juice	Tea sweetened with stevia
Fruit	Lemons, Limes, Berries
Soy Sauce	Coconut Aminos
Sugar or Artificial Sweeteners	Stevia, Xylitol, Monk Fruit or Erythritol
Vegetable Cooking Oils	Ghee, Coconut Oil or Avocado Oil
Alcohol, Beer, or Wine	Kombucha

FAT-BURNING FOODS

The opposite of fat storing is fat burning. You now know how your body stores fat, so now let's look at how it burns fat.

All the food you consume, be it carbs or protein, eventually breaks down into glucose. The body needs glucose to survive as glucose is your body's fuel source. If it can get glucose immediately out of the bloodstream, it prefers to do that instead of using up the reserved fat stores.

Fats are a rich source of energy for the body, yielding more than twice the energy on a per-weight basis as carbohydrates. This is why fat is the body's preferred fuel for survival and it doesn't give it up willingly. Your body prefers to burn carbohydrates and store fat in preparation for a threat of starvation. In order to achieve weight loss though, we do not want the body to operate in this manner.

Our objective is to burn fat, so we want our body to have to go into the fat cells and use that for fuel instead of just constantly burning carbohydrates that came from your last meal. Here is how we make that happen. When the body needs glucose and there isn't enough in the bloodstream (from eating a high-carbohydrate meal), the pancreas is signaled to release the hormone *glucagon*. Glucagon stimulates the release of glycogen (stored glucose) from fat storage to be used up for energy. This is how fat burning occurs.

Think of glucagon as the key that goes into the fat cell, unlocks the fat, and sends it to the muscle site to be burned by the muscle. Glucagon first depletes the glucose in the muscle cells, then the liver cells, then finally in the fat cells. This is why it takes at least three days to get into true fat-burning mode, and once you are there, you'll want to stay there to get the most fat burning accomplished possible.

Another way we can lose weight 3X faster is by taking advantage of prime-time fat burning. This is important to note. If you go too long without eating or don't eat the right foods, your body will not release glucagon and you will not burn fat. Instead, because of the drop in blood sugar levels (also known as a crash), your body will burn muscle instead of fat. It is important to eat the right types of food at the right times throughout the day to prevent the spikes and the drops in blood sugar levels. The trick is keeping the levels in check throughout the day so that maximum fat burning can occur.

The chart below is a great reference point of how your body reacts to consuming specific foods as well as skipping meals or not consuming enough calories.

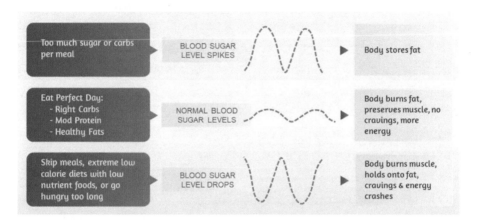

The cause and effect of each action may be a lot to remember, so if nothing else please etch the following into your memory: Whatever you do, do not skip meals! Skipping meals causes the body to release stress hormones like cortisol and then insulin. This combo puts the body into muscle-burning instead of fat-burning mode. Skipping meals also causes an imbalance in brain chemistry that leads to binge eating later in the day.

Has this ever happened to you? You are so busy throughout the day that you forget to eat and then come dinnertime, you eat everything on the table and in the pantry, then can't seem to quit snacking until you go to bed? It's definitely happened to me more than once.

So while you think you're helping yourself to eat less, you're actually causing yourself to lose weight slower and burn the wrong component of your body! This is why low-calorie diets and other starvation diets do not work.

I want to make a quick note about intermittent fasting. This is an advanced technique to take your fitness and health to the next level and in my opinion, should only be used after you've gone through the 3X Weight Loss Program and lost the majority of your weight. It is something I recommend in additional phases of 3X Weight Loss, after you have optimized your metabolism and have handled any nutritional deficiencies or hormonal imbalances. Intermittent fasting is not something you should just jump into willy-nilly before your body is ready for it. The 3X Weight Loss protocol is the safest first step approach to losing weight quickly and fasting is not necessary or recommended at this point.

THE 3X MEAL PLAN

So what is the perfect diet? It seems that everyone out there has a different opinion about what a healthy diet is. If you asked a 100 people what it means to eat healthily, you would get 100 different answers. And to make matters worse, the so-called experts themselves all have different opinions.

What is so amazing about this program is that the advice is scientific and proven to work; it is not just a gimmick or temporary weight-loss solution. As a result, this plan will become your blueprint for life. It was designed for real-life, busy women, so you can let out a sigh of relief that when I say that you won't even have to think about the steps you'll be taking!

This is the meal plan for weight loss, but it's also a plan for optimal health. You'll never have to wonder what you should eat again; this is all you will ever need. No more guessing, no more jumping from diet plan to diet plan. And once you start, you won't want to stop. It truly becomes a normal part of your everyday routine.

As a reminder, the 3X Meal Plan has been specially developed so that you burn the most fat in the shortest time with the least effort. It was created in a way that keeps your blood sugar levels normal throughout the day so that you aren't storing fat and that you actually burn fat, not muscle. It also works to promote a healthy gut so that you can actually digest your food properly and absorb the nutrients that you eat. Because food, no matter how healthy it is, is only as good as you can absorb and assimilate it. You could have the most perfect diet at your fingertips but if you have digestive issues like reflux, gas, constipation, bloating, or diarrhea, then your digestive system is not functioning correctly, and you won't be adequately getting nutrients from the food you are eating.

The 3X Meal Plan not only provides the body with the essential nutrients that your metabolism needs to function optimally, but it also eliminates cravings for sugar and junk food, keeping and you full and satisfied without feeling hungry throughout the day. In fact, the biggest challenge I have with the majority of women on this plan is that they aren't hungry at all and I have to constantly remind them to eat to make sure they stay in fat-burning mode.

The 3X meal plan is a "clean food" program made up of wholesome, preferably organic, unprocessed foods with a combination of protein, fat-burning carbs, and healthy fats.

Let's now jump in and explore the ins and outs of it!

ORGANIC FOODS

Though organic foods are often perceived as just a more expensive type of food, there is so much more to them than their price point. Organic foods are grown without the use of pesticides, synthetic fertilizers, or genetically modified organisms. Additionally, animals that produce meat, poultry, eggs, and dairy products do not eat genetically altered foods, take antibiotics, or growth hormones.

Let's now look at it from the opposite lens: If you don't eat organic, even though it may be cheaper, you are eating food that has been sprayed with highly toxic pesticides and synthetic fertilizers, fed antibiotics, and pumped with growth hormones. You will also be eating foods that were made with GMOs and sprayed with glyphosate.

Pesticides and growth hormones that are used in the production of non-organic food **severely alter** your metabolism by hijacking your hormonal system. Remember earlier when I discussed endocrine disruptors? The pesticides used on non-organic food is a known endocrine disruptor and major cause of hormonal imbalances. So if you have a thyroid issue or any other metabolic or hormonal imbalance, switching to an organic diet is the best thing you can do for your hormone health.

The first thing I usually hear when I tell a client to switch to an organic diet is that she can't afford it. In my opinion, this is just a matter of viewpoint. When you know what's at stake and you know what cheap, toxic food does to your health, then it's easier to put things into perspective. Organic food costs a lot less than expensive doctor visits or hospital bills as a result of not taking the best care of yourself. Instead of insurance I call it "ENSURE-ANCE" because you are ensuring you will have the best chance at good health and less costs on healthcare bills. If you make your health a priority you can most certainly find other areas of your life that aren't as important as your health that you are spending money on. From there you can reallocate your budget towards affording healthier food.

Most women balk at the idea of spending money on organic food at first. But they soon realize that once they get rid of all the other junk that they used to buy, they actually save money on the 3X program even while eating organic because they are no longer buying all the "filler" foods and snacks that they used to. Also, you will not eat out nearly as much, so you will save a lot of money in that regard as well.

For instance, one large (non-organic dinner salad at a typical restaurant costs anywhere from $17-$23. Once you add tax and tip on top of that you've spent around $30 for one meal! My meals prepared at home, even though they are 100% organic, average $3-$5 per meal. I am actually saving money and eating much higher quality food when eating at home.

If up until now you've thought it would be impossible to eat organic on a budget, I have good news for you: It's probably much easier than you previously thought. In fact, you could already be shopping at stores that sell affordable, organic foods at competitive prices without even realizing it. While you can shop at your local health food store, I'm pleased to say that in this day and age, there are many other options. Take Wal-Mart for example. They've started carrying all kinds of organic foods at pennies more than their non-organic counterparts. If you shop at Wal-Mart regularly like more than half of Americans, finding organic food there will be a no-brainer. You just have to know what to look for.

Organic foods sold at Wal-Mart include: eggs, olive oil, mustard, apple cider vinegar, garbanzo beans, iceberg lettuce, baby carrots, avocados, spinach, and much more! Typically, you can find the organic options stocked next to the non-organic versions. Kudos to Wal-Mart for bringing these affordable options to the masses!

Costco also has a great selection of organic foods. There, you canfind organic produce, sauerkraut, frozen vegetables, eggs, grass-fed beef, wild-caught Alaskan salmon and dozens of other items at competitive prices. Since Costco changes their selection on a regular basis, it's always fun to see what "new" organic items they have. But your options don't stop at Wal-Mart and Costco. Trader Joe's and Target sell organic foods as well. So, if you have been shopping at any of these major chains, start looking around for their affordable organic foods – you may be surprised at what you find!

ORDERING HEALTHY FOOD ONLINE

For those of you who may not have convenient access to the aforementioned stores or prefer delivery services, there are options for you as well. Thanks to modern technology, you can shop for organic products from the comfort of your living room.

Nowadays, we can get our grocery shopping done in ten minutes flat without putting on makeup or leaving the house! Not only that, but when you buy your favorite organic foods online, you can save a ton of money in the process, slashing your grocery bill every month. There are lots of places you can order organic food online, such as www.thrivemarket.com, www.vitacost.com, www.uswellnessmeats.com, www.sunfood.com, and www.forthegourmet.com.

You can also opt for a food delivery service that shops and prepares all your food for you and delivers it straight to your doorstep. My personal favorite is www.greenchef.com.

SHOPPING AT FARMER'S MARKETS

In addition to large chains and online grocers, you can also get amazing organic food at your local farmer's market. While the selections vary, you can often find fruits, vegetables, organic eggs, locally grown honey, nuts, cheeses, and meats at farmer's markets. Even if the food isn't certified organic (because it's such an expensive process), it's usually pesticide-free.

I also love how you can meet the farmer personally and speak to them about their practices. You can ask them if they use herbicides and pesticides, what their chickens eat, and if their cows roam free and eat grass in the pasture. For example, I was at a farmer's market once and I noticed a man selling wild-caught salmon. He gave me all the details on how the fish was caught, where it came from, and how they packed and shipped it to maintain freshness and taste. He quickly sold me on his process and quality.

He told me how the salmon is caught out in the ocean and then brought back to the dock where it is immediately cut up and flash frozen on the spot. He got me excited about the amazing process, so I purchased a couple pounds of frozen salmon. It was the best salmon I ever tasted. I ended up getting his phone number and now I meet up with him a couple times a year to buy salmon from him in bulk.

BUYING FROM FARMERS AND RANCHERS DIRECT

We eat a lot of eggs in our family and since we want the highest quality eggs (pasture-raised, organic, and soy-free), we decided it would be more cost-effective to find a local farmer who sold eggs. We found a guy who sells eggs from chickens who roam free and eat grass and vegetable scraps (the things they're supposed to eat); happy chickens! Now we buy our eggs from him instead of buying them at a grocery store.

My husband and I purchase a cow from a local farmer each year and we end up paying about $4.00 a pound. It isn't certified organic, but we personally know the farmer. His cows graze on their ten-acre property eating grass in the sunlight twelve months out of the year. We know that we are getting really good, high-quality, 100% grass-fed meat for less than what conventionally grain-fed cows cost at a grocery store.

Our beef, salmon, and eggs all come from local vendors. We end up paying less money for very high-quality food and in turn, we're supporting our local farmers. You can go to www.eatwild.com to find local pasture-based farms and ranches in your area that produce grass-fed eggs, meat, and dairy products. If you can't find what you're looking for locally, Eatwild also has a list of farms that will ship directly to your door.

Another great resource is the National Farmers Market Directory from the United States Department of Agriculture (www.ams.usda.gov/local-food-directories/farmersmarkets). Once on the site, you simply enter your state and the USDA will generate a list of all the farmer's markets in your state. It doesn't get easier than that!

I've mentioned supporting local farmers a few times now, but why? It's important to support your local farmers for several reasons. For starters, locally-grown food is better for your body. The less time between the farm and the table, the more nutrient-dense the food is. When produce is shipped, or imported from far away, it's picked before it's ripe. Then, it travels miles on trucks and planes and sits in a warehouse before it makes it to the supermarket, let alone your table. Locally-grown crops, on the other hand, are picked at the peak of perfection, so you benefit from all of the nutrients and it tastes much better. Additionally, the price you pay at a farmer's market is low because farmers are cutting the middleman out. You pay wholesale prices while supporting the farmers' families and the community as a whole. It's a win-win situation.

Buying local food also preserves open space so farmers aren't forced to sell their land to big developers. When you buy locally grown produce, meats, and dairy, you're doing your part to support local families, to benefit the environment and wildlife, to protect precious water sources, and to conserve fertile soil. I could go on and on about the benefits of supporting your local farmers, so let's just say that by supporting your local farmers, you're helping to ensure that these small farms will be in your community for generations to come.

Now that you know the quality of food that you should eat on the 3X program, let's transition now into discussing the different types of food you should eat.

PROTEIN

One of the most important food groups is protein. Protein is what provides your body with the tools (amino acids) it needs to build and repair your organs, tissues, muscles, and bones. The breaking down and repairing of different body parts is an ongoing process that your body goes through daily. So without sufficient protein, your body will break down muscle in order to get what it needs for more important functions like your heart and your lungs.

The breakdown of muscle is something you absolutely do not want because muscle mass is what burns fat. We want to make sure we maintain the muscle mass that you currently have through getting adequate amounts of high-quality, usable protein, and then once you've lost your excess body fat, you'll want to focus on strengthening and building your muscles with exercise so that you can continue to burn fat long term.

This is another big problem I've noticed with other diet programs, lack of emphasis on the importance of getting enough protein. Again, if one is focused solely on calories they will inevitably neglect the source of the calories and be doing their metabolism a serious dis-favor.

Furthermore, increasing protein along with fiber elevates the fat-burning hormone glucagon, while lowering the fat-storing hormone insulin. This hormonal balancing effect enhances the utilization of fat and produces what is known as the thermic effect of food. This is an increased period of calorie burning induced by foods with extra protein and fiber that stimulate extra fat burning to take place.

You need to have a selection of protein with each meal of the day.

FAT-BURNING CARBS & VEGETABLES

To eat carbs or not to eat carbs: That is the question. Carbohydrates are easy-to-use fuels. This means that when you eat carbs your body uses them up quickly for energy. That sounds like a good thing, right? Well here's the kicker (there's always a kicker): Any leftover carbs in your bloodstream immediately get stored as fat.

The double whammy is that when your body is busy consistently burning off carbs (if you eat too many or the wrong ones) it does not ever tap into fat storage. Not good if you are overweight and want to shed some pounds. Carbs *are* required to supply your body with energy, but where you get those carbohydrates from will either make or break your weight-loss results.

The carbs that are used in this program in the fat-burning phase are going to come from vegetable sources because they provide your body with energy, as well as the essential nutrients that your metabolism needs, yet they do not contain a high amount of sugar that will cause your body to store fat. They have the least effect on your blood sugar levels while providing your body with the most dense nutrition possible.

Dense nutrition is a term used to describe the concept of getting the most value out of the food you eat. Vegetables not only provide your body with fiber and fat-burning carbs, but with the vitamins, minerals, enzymes, and antioxidants your metabolism needs to properly do its job.

One thing that is very important is to know is that "weight" is a combination of body fat and water retention. When you start to lose weight, you will be losing body fat and water weight. If you are losing body fat but retaining water, it will not show up on the scale and you will begin to get discouraged thinking that you are not getting results. So it is very important to make sure you do not retain water while you are losing fat. The way you do this is by getting adequate amounts of potassium from vegetables. Sometimes it can take up to 6 months to replenish the potassium levels inside the cells. This is why I recommend eating a lot of vegetables and drinking a morning green juice every single day. Potassium not only handles water weight issues, but it also helps lower the fat-storing hormone insulin. Without getting enough potassium, you could have higher amounts of insulin in your body, which will keep you from burning fat.

Vegetables also provide your body with something called chlorophyll. Chlorophyll helps eliminate cravings, detoxes the body, helps control blood sugar levels, lowers inflammation, and melts fat.

I recommend eating an abundance of vegetables with every meal. You can have as many non-starchy vegetables as you want. Starchy vegetables are things like potatoes, French fries, hash browns, etc. Corn, by the way, is not a vegetable, but a grain. Additional fat-burning carbs are listed in the approved foods list in the pages to come.

HEALTHY FATS

Now, we've all heard that fat is bad for us, but how bad is it? Are all fats the same?

No, they are not. Bad fats are the ones I mentioned in the previous section. Things like vegetable oils and trans fats definitely need to be avoided. However, not all fats are created equal.

When it comes to your health, there are some important points to know about fat. First, your brain is 60% fat and requires fat to work properly. Secondly, each one of your cells is wrapped in a layer of fat and it depends on it to keep the nutrients in the cell and toxins out of your cells.

Furthermore, your body needs fat to manufacture hormones. Your entire body is run by your hormonal system, so having it work properly is pretty important. Fats are a vital nutrient for your body and despite what you have heard in the past, fat does not make you overweight as long as you avoid the bad ones and eat the right ones.

So you will want to include at least one tablespoon of healthy fats per meal and eat even more throughout the day if needed. And if you ever feel hungry or start to have cravings, just know that you need more healthy fats, not a Snickers bar.

Just for reference, when you cook with oil, the best oil to use is avocado oil. It has the highest smoke point and can withstand higher temperatures than most other oils. The next best oils for cooking are animal fat, ghee, coconut oil, and palm oil. I wouldn't heat olive oil or other nut or seed oils because they are very fragile oils and can break down in the heating process. Heat changes the molecular structure of the oils, which creates damaging free radicals.

FAT-BURNING FOOD LIST

I personally spent over a year perfecting this plan and hand selected the absolute BEST foods that help you burn fat FAST so that you can make quick meals without being hungry, fighting cravings, or feeling deprived!

This list of foods takes the guesswork out of what to make for each meal and gives you exactly the foods to eat that will give you weight-loss results that will last.

Here is a list of approved foods on the 3X Program:

Protein

- ☐ Organic Chicken
- ☐ Organic Eggs (preferably soy-free)
- ☐ Organic Turkey
- ☐ Organic Grass-fed Beef
- ☐ Grass-fed Bison
- ☐ Venison
- ☐ Lamb
- ☐ Duck
- ☐ Wild Fish (Salmon, Trout, Halibut, Tuna, Sardines, Anchovies, etc.)
- ☐ Wild Shellfish (Crab, Oysters, Shrimp, Clams, Mussels, Scallops)

Vegetables

- ☐ All Herbs and Spices
- ☐ Artichokes
- ☐ Asparagus
- ☐ Arugula
- ☐ Avocado
- ☐ Bamboo Shoots
- ☐ Bean Sprouts
- ☐ Beets
- ☐ Greens
- ☐ Brussels Sprouts
- ☐ Broccoli
- ☐ Bell Peppers
- ☐ Bok Choy
- ☐ Cabbage
- ☐ Carrots
- ☐ Cassava (use sparingly)
- ☐ Cauliflower
- ☐ Celery
- ☐ Chard
- ☐ Chicory greens
- ☐ Chili peppers
- ☐ Collard Greens
- ☐ Cucumbers
- ☐ Dill Pickles
- ☐ Dulse
- ☐ Eggplant
- ☐ Endive
- ☐ Escarole
- ☐ Fennel
- ☐ Fermented Vegetables
- ☐ Green Beans
- ☐ Green Leafy Lettuces (all kinds)
- ☐ Hearts of Palm
- ☐ Jicama (raw)
- ☐ Kale
- ☐ Kimchi
- ☐ Leeks
- ☐ Mushrooms
- ☐ Olives

- ☐ Onions
- ☐ Radicchio
- ☐ Seaweed
- ☐ Sauerkraut
- ☐ Snap Peas
- ☐ Snow Peas
- ☐ Spinach
- ☐ Sprouts
- ☐ Squash
- ☐ Sweet Potatoes
- ☐ Tomatoes
- ☐ Turnip Greens
- ☐ Watercress
- ☐ Yams
- ☐ Zucchini

Fruit

- ☐ Berries (Blackberries, blueberries, raspberries, strawberries)
- ☐ Lemons
- ☐ Limes

Healthy Fats

- ☐ Avocado Oil
- ☐ Cacao Butter
- ☐ Coconut Butter
- ☐ Coconut Oil
- ☐ Extra Virgin Olive Oil
- ☐ Grass-fed Ghee
- ☐ Grass-Fed Meat Fat
- ☐ Hazelnut Oil
- ☐ Hemp Seed Oil
- ☐ Macadamia Nut Oil
- ☐ Palm Oil
- ☐ Sesame Seed Oil
- ☐ Walnut Oil

Nuts/Seeds (Preferably Sprouted)

- ☐ Almonds
- ☐ Walnuts
- ☐ Cashews
- ☐ Brazil Nuts
- ☐ Sunflower Seeds
- ☐ Pumpkin Seeds
- ☐ Chia Seeds

Misc. Fat Burning Carbs

- ☐ Quinoa
- ☐ Garbanzo Beans
- ☐ Sweet Potatoes
- ☐ Cassava
- ☐ Tapioca

Misc. Condiments

- ☐ Organic Chicken Stock
- ☐ Organic Vegetable Stock
- ☐ Organic Beef Stock
- ☐ Mustard
- ☐ Sea Salt
- ☐ Coconut Aminos (replaces soy sauce)
- ☐ Coconut Flour
- ☐ Almond Flour
- ☐ Coconut Milk
- ☐ Coconut Vinegar
- ☐ Apple Cider Vinegar
- ☐ Red Wine Vinegar
- ☐ Frank's Hot Sauce
- ☐ Primal Kitchen Avocado Oil Mayo

Beverages

- ☐ Almond Milk
- ☐ Cashew Milk
- ☐ Coconut Milk
- ☐ Sparkling Mineral Water
- ☐ Spring Water
- ☐ Kombucha
- ☐ Organic Coffee
- ☐ Organic Tea

Sweeteners

- ☐ Stevia
- ☐ Xylitol
- ☐ Monk Fruit
- ☐ Erythritol
- ☐ Raw Cacao Nibs
- ☐ Raw Cocoa Powder

CHAPTER 6

THE 7 DAILY FAT-BURNING ACTIVITIES

THE PERFECT DAY

When I was trying to lose weight, I was very frustrated with all the random, confusing, unorganized pieces of information out there about what to eat to lose weight. Every diet was so different from the next and I felt so confused not knowing what to trust. Thus, I ended up trying so many programs before creating 3X.

Prior to 3X, if I had a bad day and cheated on the diet, I felt like a failure and completely gave up. From there it was on to the next tip, fad, or gimmick. I was constantly yo-yoing and never got close to reaching my goal.

I'm a busy mom of two young children and do not have time for crazy, complex diets that require doing three different phases of cleanses, detoxes, and "resets." I just couldn't keep up with things like measuring out my food or calculating out the ratios between carbs, fat, and protein. I also did not have time to spend hours of my day cooking in the kitchen.

I wanted a program that was simple but with enough flexibility so that I would never get bored with my food and could still enjoy my life. I wanted a proven blueprint or template that if followed, would actually get me results. Not something that would work sometimes for some people, but a 100-percent, dialed-in plan that had a known and guaranteed predictable outcome. Not something that I would have to "go on," which meant I would come off. I wanted a lifelong, healthy lifestyle plan that would help me lose weight and was realistic to do every day of my life, even after I lost all my of weight.

What I was searching for was The Perfect Day, a daily checklist of the exact things I needed to do daily to be the healthiest version of me. When I realized that what I was looking for didn't exist, I knew I had to create it. But let me tell you, it wasn't easy. Sifting through all the false information and going through the hundreds of weight-loss programs to try to figure out all the right things to do to achieve a perfect state of balance (homeostasis) to get the fastest results possible was quite an undertaking.

I first had to learn how the body worked so that I knew what it needed to be in balance. Then I had to figure out exactly what foods to eat and what foods not to eat.

Next, I had to determine how to eat healthy, yet feel satisfied so that I didn't feel hungry or have cravings. I knew from previous experience when trying to eat healthy that if I felt hungry or had cravings for unhealthy food, I would cave into it and fall off track.

From there, I had to develop a system so that I could make it all simple and easy to follow in order to save time each day. I'm a busy mom with a household, a husband, kids to take care of, and a business to run, and I don't have time for complex dieting techniques or to go to the gym every night and do hours of cardio.

Not only that, but I had to learn how to get motivated when I was feeling low and had to learn how to keep myself accountable so that I would stay on track and continue to reach my goal weight. It was a really hard process and took me almost an entire year of full-time research to place all the pieces of the puzzle.

I can now proudly say that it has been not only created, but continues to be used by thousands of women around the world who have completely changed their health and their body with this simple, proven daily checklist. The perfect, healthy lifestyle plan that works **100% of the time with everyone who uses it**: The Perfect Day.

The 3X Weight Loss Perfect Day is a daily checklist that you follow to have the most perfect day of optimum health and weight loss. This includes what foods to eat, what foods to avoid, what supplements to take, how much water to drink, what kind of exercises to do, and how much sleep to get, all laid out into a simple, step-by-step routine.

The best part about The Perfect Day is that it's an exact blueprint that if followed, will get you to your goal weight. If you end up cheating or going off the program, you'll know exactly what to do to get back on. You'll never have to guess or wonder what to do or what to eat because you know with certainty that The Perfect Day is your go-to fat burning plan. *This* is your roadmap to reaching your goal weight and following it every day is the fastest way to get the body you want.

Here's another success story that I'd like to share with you. Andrea N. started the program on 12/29/2016. As of 8/1/17, in just 7 months, she has lost 76 pounds, 41 total inches, 17% body fat, and five dress sizes.

I started my weight-loss journey after I had struggled with my weight for over 12 years. I had been an athlete in high school and received my Bachelor's degree in Athletic Training, so I had the knowledge base on nutrition and fitness. My weight became a problem in my late twenties when I met my husband

and started having children. My body was changing, but my eating habits were not.

I would do Weight Watchers, South Beach, and Paleo. Each time I would lose 10-15 pounds but put it right back on when I would get frustrated or stressed with not losing more weight. I slowly kept packing on pounds, wishing that I could do something to get them off. My mindset about food changed. I looked to eat when I was stressed, happy, sad, or bored.

My breaking point was when I turned 39 the summer of 2016. I was at the heaviest I had ever been. I would not take pictures with my kids because I was ashamed of how I looked. I wanted to get serious about losing weight, but again did not have the tools or a plan on how to do this. I thought I would work out and count calories. By late fall of 2016, I was not losing anything and my deadline of losing 80 pounds by August of 2017 was slipping away. I started looking into the gastric sleeve with my primary care physician and insurance when I saw my aunt who had lost 40 pounds in a four-month period. She told me about the 3X Program and said when I was ready to commit to losing weight to get a hold of her and she would get me some info.

My husband asked what I wanted for Christmas. I told him I wanted to lose weight and to do the 3X Program. My journey began on December 29, 2016 with 100% support from him.

The 3X Program equipped me with the knowledge that I never got with any other weight-loss program that I had tried. The Academy (inside the 3X Weight Loss Video Coaching program) changed my thought process on food and made me realize what I was putting in my mouth not only caused me to gain weight, but was making me sick. That alone, for me, was motivation to stay on track.

When I would want to cheat, I made myself review the lessons in the academy in my head or even pull out the computer and look at it again. When the scale started moving in the right direction, it gave me more motivation to stay on track and keep following The Perfect Day. I lost more weight in one month on 3X than I did with any other program that I would follow for months on end. In seven short months, I reached my goal of losing the weight (76 pounds) before I turned 40!

I am a creature of habit. I make sure that my husband and I meal prep on Sundays to make it easy for us to stay on track through the week. I used to eat out for lunch every day because that was the easiest thing for me to do while working. I now grab protein out of my fridge that we grill on Sunday, my salad full of greens and veggies, and I am set for lunch. We follow the recipes on the 3X Program for dinners and I definitely use the knowledge that is on the 3X Facebook page of ideas as well. Now that I am at my goal weight, I step on the scale 2 days a week to make sure that I am staying on track.

We had a big birthday month that came with cake, eating out, and parties. For the most part, I stayed on track, but did partake in some of the festivities. The scale moved a couple of pounds up, but as soon as I got back to my perfect days and tightened the "ropes," I was right back where I needed to be. That eased my mind in knowing that I can have a day where I might not follow the program 100%, but as long as I get back to the basics all will be good.

Thank you, Laura, for this program. It has changed my life!

-Andrea N.

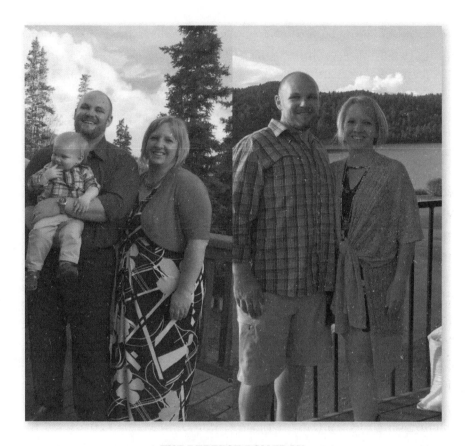

THE PERFECT DAY PLAN
FAT-BURNING ACTION #1: JUICING

According to the CDC, less than one-third of adult Americans eat the recommended nine servings of vegetables a day. This is why I recommend starting each morning with a fresh green vegetable juice. It is the most effective way to get vegetables into your body and to virtually guarantee that you will reach your daily target in an easily digestible form.

Not to mention the morning is prime time for nutrient absorption because your body is in a fasting state due to not having any food for 10 or more hours. Additionally, the first thing you put into your body in the morning is very important because you are going to utilize those nutrients better than any other time.

When you drink fresh-pressed vegetable juice, it bypasses the digestive process and the nutrients go straight into your bloodstream and into your cells, all within a matter of minutes. Green vegetable juice is chock full of the essential micronutrients that are vital for the metabolism to run optimally. Outside of taking supplements, drinking green vegetable juice in the morning is the most efficient way to get those much-needed nutrients into your body as quickly as possible.

Juicing has also been shown to have great effects for weight loss. In one study, adults who drank at least eight ounces of vegetable juice as part of a diet lost four pounds over 12 weeks, while those who followed the same diet but did not drink the juice lost only one pound. The vegetable juice drinkers also significantly increased their intake of vitamin C and potassium levels.

Fresh green vegetable juice is loaded with potassium and will help you with water retention issues and to lower the fat-storing hormone insulin.

Most women love the green juice and they look forward to drinking it every single morning. However, if you've never juiced, then it may be an initial shock to your system. If this is the case, start out slow with just cucumbers, celery, a little bit of lemon, and ginger and then add on more green vegetables from there as you get used it.

Believe it or not, sooner or later your body will begin to crave the green juice and you will begin to love it. The green juice is a vital part of the program. It keeps your body alkalized, helps with digestion, speeds your metabolism, nourishes your cells, and will help eliminate cravings and hunger throughout the day.

I recommend using a juicer, but if you only have a blender then you can blend the vegetables and strain out the pulp. But just know that juicing tastes a lot better than blending. If blending, you will have to find a combination of vegetables that work for you because blending has a completely different taste and texture than juicing. I prefer juicing and do not like blending my vegetables, but you can do whatever works for you! Do not add fruits, carrots, or beets, because once they are juiced they are just pure sugar, which will keep you from burning fat.

If you are traveling and cannot juice fresh, then you can purchase an organic green juice powder. This definitely does not replace fresh juice but if you are in a pinch, it is the next best thing. You can also purchase pre-made juices from Whole Foods or other health food stores. Just read the ingredients carefully and don't buy any that have fruit or any kind of sugar in them.

Here is a recipe for green juice if you are using a juicer:

Organic ingredients only

- ☐ 2 kale leaves with stem
- ☐ 1 collard green leaf (or other dark leafy greens)
- ☐ 2 celery stalks
- ☐ ½ large cucumber
- ☐ 1 large juiced lemon
- ☐ Parsley and cilantro
- ☐ Pinch of salt
- ☐ Pinch of cayenne pepper

I highly recommend reading the book *The Rainbow Juice Cleanse* by Dr. Ginger Southall, for more information and recipes about juicing for weight loss.

FAT-BURNING ACTION #2: MEALS

You can breathe a sigh of relief because this program is simple and does not require you to count calories, measure portions, or do any other complex method of dieting, nor do you have to kill yourself in the gym to lose weight. All you have to do is eat foods that burn fat and don't eat foods that store fat.

Each meal in the 3X Program is made up of protein, carbohydrates, and healthy fats. It is very important that you get all three of these components in each meal because they work together to nourish your body, help you burn fat, prevent muscle loss, and keep you full and satiated throughout the day.

Let's start with breakfast.

You've heard it over and over again: Breakfast is the most important meal of the day. But what most people don't know is that it's not just breakfast that is important; it's **what you eat** for breakfast that's important. Again, this is because breakfast sets the pace of your metabolism for the entire day and what you choose for breakfast will either make or break your weight-loss efforts.

According to Byron J. Richards, Board Certified Clinical Nutritionist, the two signs of a poor breakfast are:

1. You are unable to make it five hours to lunch without food cravings or your energy crashing.
2. You are much more prone to strong food cravings later that afternoon or evening.

Do either of these sound familiar?

It pains me to see how many women suffer through diets and exhausting themselves at the gym just to have all of their hard work undone by eating the wrong breakfast.

Most women are rushed in the mornings and either skip breakfast or opt for a quick fix like a cup of coffee, some yogurt, a little fruit, a smoothie, a bar, or a muffin. This is one of the biggest diet disasters and weight loss mistakes that I see women make.

It doesn't matter how much you exercise, it's all for naught if your body is in fat-storing mode. Breakfast options that contain high levels of carbs and hidden sugars slow the metabolism, turn on fat-storing hormones, and create hunger and cravings throughout the day.

So yes, breakfast is the most important meal of the day. But what is the perfect breakfast for weight loss and fat burning? High protein! Eating a high-protein breakfast can increase your metabolism by 30% for the entire day, which is the metabolic equivalent of going on a two-to-three-mile jog! Eating a high-carbohydrate breakfast like fruit or oatmeal on the other hand, can only enhance your metabolism by 4% or less.

The perfect breakfast, in addition to being high-protein, would also consist of a healthy fat and a glass of fresh green vegetable juice for optimum nourishment and fat burning throughout the day.

Example of The Perfect Breakfast:

- ☐ Two eggs (protein) cooked any style in coconut oil or grass-fed ghee (healthy fats)
- ☐ A side of turkey bacon or chicken sausage (more protein)
- ☐ A couple slices of avocado on the side (optional)
- ☐ Glass of green vegetable juice

You could also skip the eggs and just have some turkey bacon, chicken sausage, or even leftovers from the night before.

LUNCH

It is really important that you include as many raw vegetables as you can into your day. As stated above, raw vegetables provide you with potassium as well as live enzymes that your metabolism needs to perform its daily tasks. When food is cooked, most nutrients are killed off and therefore you are not able to get the vital nutrients that are contained within the veggies.

For lunch I recommend making a huge "3X salad" with at least 3 cups of raw vegetables and dark leafy greens. You may use other toppings such as avocado, seeds, hummus, olives, pickles, etc.

Next, add your choice of protein (meat, fish, eggs, or vegetarian protein). Include a homemade dressing made with walnut, olive, or avocado oil and lemon, vinegar, herbs, and spices. My favorite is the 3X Healthy Ranch Dressing:

3X Healthy Ranch Dressing

Ingredients:

- ½ Cup Walnut Oil
- 1/4 Cup Pickle Juice (I use Bubbie's)
- 1/8 Cup Apple Cider Vinegar
- 1/4 Cup Pumpkin Seeds
- 1 TBSP Sea Salt
- 1 TBSP Black Pepper
- 1 Garlic Clove

Directions: Place all ingredients in a high-speed blender for minimum of 30 seconds or until desired consistency is achieved. A video tutorial can be found here: https://3xweightloss.com/dairy-free-healthy-ranch-dressing.

I also highly recommend adding ½ cup of sauerkraut to your salad.

Let's discuss sauerkraut for a minute because it's one of my "secret" weight-loss weapons and it deserves special mention. It plays a significant role in fat burning and is a very valuable tool for your healthy lifestyle toolbox.

Merriam-Webster defines sauerkraut as: "Cabbage cut fine and fermented in a brine made of its own juice with salt." German for "sour greens," sauerkraut takes cabbage, one of the healthiest foods on the planet, and combines it with fermentation, which is one of the most beneficial food preparation methods in existence.

Sauerkraut's first known use was in 1617 in Eastern Europe, but it didn't make its way to North America until the 1700s when immigrants brought it over on ships. Because it was fermented, lasted a long time, and was chock full of nutrients, sauerkraut travelled well on long journeys from Europe to the U.S.

Why is fermented cabbage so beneficial? The fermentation process produces gut-friendly probiotics, which are your body's first line of defense against toxins and harmful bacteria that enter your body. Studies found that good bacteria are critical for lowering the risk of virtually every medical condition and chronic illness under the sun, including cancer, food allergies, autoimmune diseases, leaky gut syndrome, brain disorders, and many more.

Foods rich in probiotics, like sauerkraut, improve immune function, aid in digestion and brain function, and reduce inflammation—one of the leading causes of acute conditions and chronic diseases. Inflammation also greatly contributes to being overweight and blocks your ability to burn fat. So anything you can do to lower inflammation is a good thing! Probiotic-rich foods offer many health benefits because they help lower the risk of a host of health problems including:

- Cancer
- Asthma
- Weight gain
- Mental illness

- Ulcerative colitis
- Digestive disorders
- Hormonal imbalances
- Depression and anxiety

Probiotic foods feed gut-friendly bacteria, decrease toxins and bad bacteria, regulate hormonal fluctuations, decrease stress, aid in digestion, improve the immune system and cognitive function, and provide cancer-fighting antioxidants. As a low-calorie, anti-inflammatory food that's rich in probiotics, vitamins C and K, calcium, potassium, and phosphorus, it's definitely worth piling this stuff on your salad every day!

SNACKS

One of my go-to snacks when I feel like having something crunchy is celery sticks with almond butter. You can also have things like nuts, vegetables dipped in hummus, turkey rolls with mustard and avocado or hard-boiled eggs.

In my opinion, protein is the best option for a snack because it helps prevent muscle loss, increases fat burning, and keeps you fuller longer. Having this as an afternoon snack not only satisfies your afternoon hunger and cravings, but also boosts your energy when you are hitting the typical afternoon slump.

DINNER

Dinner should be your lightest meal of the day and you should try to eat dinner three hours before bed to burn the most fat while you sleep. The meal should be comprised of a protein (meat, fish, eggs, or vegetarian protein) with three or more cups of raw or cooked vegetables and a healthy fat.

FAT-BURNING ACTION #3: SUPPLEMENTS

In my work as a weight-loss coach, I have found that one-for-one, my clients who were deficient in particular nutrients found their bodies to be very stubborn about releasing stored body fat. I can't stress enough how important it is on a weight-loss program to replenish and repair yourself with an abundance of nutrients. It is really hard to get all of the nutrients that your body needs to safely and rapidly burn fat solely from food, which is why I recommend supplements to go along with the program.

In my opinion, supplementing with good, high-quality vitamins and minerals is the fastest way to help repair a stalled, or even "dead," metabolism. I have found several supplements to be the most helpful to weight loss and recommend them to be taken as part of this program. But before I tell you which supplements I recommend, it's important that you know how to choose a good-quality supplement.

CHOOSING QUALITY SUPPLEMENTS

Now that you understand why it's important to take supplements for optimal health and weight loss, let's discuss how to choose the best type, because not all supplements are created equal.

Going in as a blind consumer, you can easily get overwhelmed and confused by the massive variety of choices you have. With no idea what makes one vitamin better than the next, it's common to just choose one because of the pretty packaging, the price, or whatever the vitamin guy in the store told you to buy. In other words, you can be put in an undesirable situation if you don't know what to look for in a vitamin.

The last thing you want to do is take a supplement that has bad, low-quality ingredients, or to spend money on a supplement that doesn't actually contain what it stated on the label. You may think that that would never happen, but I assure you, it does.

As a matter of fact, in 2015 the New York State Attorney General's office conducted an investigation into top-selling store brands of herbal supplements at four national retailers and found that they were grossly mislabeled. Supplements that were labeled as gluten free had wheat in them, supplements that were labeled "Gingko Biloba" contained no gingko at all, etc. As they continued their tests, they actually found that four out of five of the products did not contain any of the herbs on their labels. So how can you be certain when you're buying supplements that you are getting what you think you're getting?

The first thing you want to do is make sure they are third-party tested and certified, because supplements are not regulated and the manufacturers can basically put whatever they want in a bottle, slap a label on it, and put it on the shelf. But if the supplement is third-party tested and certified by an organization such as National Science Foundation (NSF), then it has been validated to contain the nutrients it states on the label.

NSF is the only American National Standard that establishes requirements for the ingredients in dietary and nutritional supplements. There are three main components of the NSF dietary supplements certification program:

- Label claim review to certify that what's on the label is in the bottle
- Toxicology review to certify product formulation
- Contaminant review to ensure the product contains no undeclared ingredients or unacceptable levels of contaminants

So, if your supplements are certified by NSF, you are safe from mislabeling.

Third-party certifications also guarantee that the product routinely proves solubility and absorption within the body, as well as purity testing according to the level that the brand is certified for.

The highest level of certification within vitamin manufacturing is the OTC level, because the precision necessary to attain and maintain this certification level is a process that is carefully monitored under the surveillance of doctors in a sterile environment. Routine inspections by outside laboratories measure batches for consistency to ensure less than 1% deviation from batch to batch.

Many retail multi-vitamin products which are not OTC certified consistently receive reprimand and are publicly called out as containing unsafe contaminants, but are still legally allowed to continue to distribute their products with no censorship or quality controls at all.

Consumers must be vigilant about their purchasing choices because **supplement manufacturers are not required by law to submit to quality inspections**, and these certifications are only pursued by companies that are interested in proving the quality of their process.

This is why it is critical to ensure that you choose a brand with effective testing and purification methods in place, as well as third-party certifications to prove ongoing efficacy and safety.

The next thing to look for in a supplement is the quality of the ingredients because even if they're certified, that does not mean that they contain ingredients from high-quality sources. The quality of the ingredients used in the supplement, just like the quality of your food, means a lot when it comes to its effectiveness inside your body.

I recommend choosing supplements that are GMO free, pesticide free, soy free, gluten free, and are whole-food based, not synthetic.

Also, you'll want to make sure they are bioavailable (meaning they can be absorbed and used by the body) and that they are in capsule, not tablet form. In order to make tablets, manufactures have to use glues, binders, and fillers and apply hundreds of thousands of pounds of pressure to keep the ingredients intact.

Because of the amount of pressure used to create tablets and how compacted the ingredients are, the body rarely ever breaks them down. Most of the time, they just pass right through without being absorbed, which means they are a complete waste of money.

Now that you have a better guideline about how to choose supplements, you can feel more confident when making your purchasing decision. If you are interested to know the exact brands I use inside the 3X Weight Loss program please visit: www.3XWeightLoss.com/supplements.

Here are the types of supplements I recommend for weight loss.

VITAMINS & MINERALS

The first is a whole-food-based multi-vitamin and mineral to give you the basic essential vitamins and minerals necessary for an optimal metabolism. When your body is deficient in nutrients, it will not want to release fat and you will most likely have cravings. Providing your body with essential vitamins and minerals can help speed your metabolism by giving it the nutrients it needs to function properly. When your body is nourished, you will not feel hungry or have to fight cravings and it will release fat more readily.

B-12

A particularly important vitamin to help with weight loss is vitamin B-12 (methylcobalamin), an essential nutrient for proper metabolism function. Use the methylated form, methylcobalamin, and not the synthetic form, which is called cyanocobalamin and is very harmful. Cyanocobalamin is a cheap, synthetic version of vitamin B-12, which is bound to a toxic, poisonous cyanide molecule. Yes, cyanide.

OMEGA-3 FISH OIL

Next, I highly recommend omega-3 fish oil, because most people have a severe imbalance of omega-6 to omega-3 oils—way too high on the omega-6 side. Too much omega-6 and not enough omega-3 causes inflammation in the body. One of the major causes of weight gain is inflammation, as it blocks your ability to burn fat. One can use omega-3 fish oils to lower inflammation so that fat burning can occur. Furthermore, fish oil has been shown to help convert fat-storing cells (known as white fat into fat burning-cells (known as brown fat In a study published in the journal *Scientific Reports*, fish oil intake reduced body weight gain and fat accumulation. You can see the access the study here: https://www.nature.com/articles/srep18013.

COENZYME Q10 UBIQUINOL

I also recommend taking something called CoQ10 (Ubiquinol). CoQ10 is used for energy production by every cell in your body, and also helps protect against cellular damage from free radicals. Ubiquinol is the reduced form of CoQ10, the effective form your body naturally uses. CoQ10 Ubiquinol is a key nutrient needed for energy production as it helps combat fatigue. The ability of the body to create CoQ10 declines as you age, making CoQ10 supplementation important, especially in individuals struggling with low energy.

CHLORELLA

Another important supplement that is particularly important for detoxification is chlorella. Chlorella is a green superfood and has a large amount of chlorophyll in it. It is a single-celled micro-algae and is so small that it can cross the blood-brain barrier and pull toxins out. It essentially helps to clean up your blood.

Chlorella is one of the best things you can do for detoxification. Studies in the *Journal of Medicinal Foods* in Japan have shown that chlorella can also help reduce body fat.

ACTIVATED CHARCOAL AND ZEOLITE

A couple of additional detox supplements I recommend are activated charcoal and zeolite. Activated charcoal is a very strong, yet safe, detoxifying agent that helps your body remove things like pesticides, insecticides, and other toxins that can interfere with normal hormone and metabolism production. Zeolite works like a sponge for heavy metals and other toxins because it is negatively charged, so heavy metals and other toxins that have a positive charge are attracted to it and then trapped and eliminated from the body.

AMINO ACIDS

Having adequate amounts of amino acids from protein in your diet is also very important for weight loss. However, protein that comes from food sources is not fully utilized by the body, making it hard to get the daily requirements of protein. Without enough protein, the body will begin to break itself down to get the amino acids it needs to build and repair body parts.

An additional type of protein that I recommend taking are branched chain amino acids. BCAA's are used often by fitness experts and athletes for their known ability to improve stamina and metabolism and help increase muscle mass and enhance weight-loss results. I definitely recommend taking branched chain amino acids (BCAA's) while on any weight-loss program.

HOMEOPATHIC REMEDIES

Homeopathy has been used for hundreds of years as a natural method to heal ailments of the body. Since the 1700's when it's use first began, thousands of homeopathic remedies have been created to treat everything from the common cold to skin disorders. Many homeopathic remedies are also believed to help increase the metabolism and relieve symptoms and factors that make it difficult to stick to a diet or exercise plan. Some homeopathic remedies can even help with things like nervousness, emotional eating and cravings. If you struggle with any of these issues, I highly recommend incorporating homeopathic remedies along with this program, as you will find that you will get faster results with less "side effects" that come from detoxing and withdrawal when first transitioning into a healthier lifestyle. Please visit www.3xweightloss.com/supplements for the specific brand of homeopathic remedies I recommend

ADAPTOGENIC HERBS

Adaptogens help the body deal with external stresses such as toxins and internal stresses like inflammation. Adaptogenic herbs work with your body to bring you back into balance.

They have been known to help with hormonal imbalances, heal the thyroid and speed up metabolism. I recommend ash-waganda root and rhodiola rosea root because they can help with the following:

- Support adrenal glands/adrenal function
- Reduce anxiety and depression
- Combat effects of stress
- Burn body fat
- Stabilize blood sugar
- Lower cholesterol
- Boost immunity

Ashwaganda root can help lower blood sugar levels, reduce cortisol (a fat storing hormone) and reduce stress within the body. It also helps with anxiety, which can lead to emotional eating and cravings. It helps stimulate thyroid function and increases insulin sensitivity, and also has anti-aging and anti-cancer properties.

Rhodiola rosea root helps with endurance and energy, mental clarity, concentration, stress, anxiety, depression, and also helps with blood sugar levels.

That's a lot of supplements, but you can see that each one has a vital part to play in a successful weight-loss program. To locate a high-quality brand of each one of them separately would be very time consuming, not to mention expensive. If you are interested in finding out more information about the exact supplements I use with the 3X Weight Loss program, please visit www.3xweightloss.com/supplements.

FAT-BURNING ACTION #4: WATER

The body is made up of 60% water. Blood is made up of 92% water. Every cell in your body is 70% water. Therefore, if you do not have adequate amount of water every function in your body will slow down (including your metabolism) and your health will begin to suffer.

The recommended daily amount of water on this program is three to four liters of water per day (there are about 34 ounces in a liter). Ideally, you will consume 1/2 of your body weight in ounces. So if you weigh 180 pounds, you should drink 90 ounces of water a day, which would be three-and-a-half liters of water.

The old saying that you only need to drink eight ounces of water a day is severely outdated and is not adequate for a rapid fat-loss routine. Water is crucial to fat loss as it helps break down and flush out fat and toxins from your system. So it is very important that you follow the recommendation above to ensure that you're giving your body the proper amount.

The body loses between ½ a liter and one liter of water each day in the simple act of exhalation. Another one to two liters of water are lost in the urine each day, and an additional 1/3 of a liter in bowel movements. You even lose water by being sedentary. Almost ½ a liter of water is lost a day in perspiration by a non-stressed patient in a hospital bed.

But not even taking exercise or diuretics into account, the daily amount of water lost by a body just in the act of living is about three liters. So if you are not replacing three liters per day at a minimum, technically you will be dehydrated. Drinking only eight cups of water each day could severely dehydrate you.

The less water you drink, the more energy that is required from food. Another interesting fact is that the sensation you get when you're thirsty and the sensation of feeling hungry are the same. So when you drink water exactly as outlined in this program, you will not get a hunger sensation until you're hungry. If you go without the water, you will get frequent hunger sensations. And yep, the sensations you felt this afternoon were because you were thirsty. Water is energy to the body, just as food is. When you get a thirsty sensation, the body is dehydrated.

Also important to note is that breaking down food requires water (the process of hydrolysis). Water breaks protein down into amino acids, fat to fatty acids, and carbs into glucose. One water molecule is required to release one fat molecule. And water is required to break down fat to be metabolized, so you lose no fat without water.

Water also activates lipase, an enzyme that breaks down fat. One liter of water activates lipase for two hours, so this is another aspect of why constant and consistent water intake is important.

For general reference, walking also stimulates lipase, low sugar activates lipase, and a rise in insulin inhibits lipase.

Water is also very important on a weight-loss program because when you gain one extra pound of fat, your body makes seven new miles of blood vessels. A person who is ten pounds overweight has 70 extra miles and a person who is 100 pounds overweight has 700 extra miles of blood vessels. Thus, the heart has to work harder and the oxygen and nutrients are dissipated due to the extra fat. The more you weigh, the more you need to drink. If you don't have enough water, then oxygen and nutrients won't get distributed adequately throughout your body.

So how much water should you drink? Three liters is the absolute minimum, but four liters is optimum. Or you can gauge it by body weight: ½ oz per pound. For example, 200 pounds = 100 ounces of water (three liters).

It is also important to note that when drinking this much water, you could also become dehydrated from mineral deficiencies. So it is vital that you are getting minerals from eating a lot of vegetables and I suggest adding real salt (sea salt onto your food or even in your water, and supplementing with additional minerals. Taking a tablespoon of apple cider vinegar daily will also help with loss of potassium which helps keep you hydrated (this also helps with muscle cramps.

I also like to use Ultima Replenisher, which you can find at Whole foods or on Amazon. I get the raspberry flavor and it adds a really nice flavor to my water and gives me an added boost of minerals and electrolytes.

FAT-BURNING ACTION #5: SLEEP

A lot of women I know disregard sleep as an important step to weight loss, but it is actually just as vital to get enough good-quality sleep as it is to remove bad food and eat good foods. You could be do everything right when it comes to losing weight, eating healthy food, avoiding bad food, drinking plenty of water and taking your supplements. However, if you are not getting good enough sleep then everything else you are doing might not be effective.

One of my clients sought my help because she was unable to lose weight no matter what she did. After looking over her current diet it seemed like she was doing everything right. I then found out she was only getting four hours of sleep per night. On top of that she was chronically stressed and constantly on the go. She was a mom and like most of us, put everybody else first. She just couldn't seem to figure out how to get more sleep.

I coached her on the importance of needing to get good sleep and that the lack of sleep was definitely the reason she wasn't losing weight. So we worked together on a plan on how she could get more sleep. I told her to take it one day at a time and just aim to go to bed earlier each night.

She made it to where she could get six hours and then finally, after a while, she was able to get seven hours of sleep each night. Just this one action *completely* changed her life. She started to see results and finally had hope that she could lose weight. But she would have never pinpointed it before because like most people, she just thought weight loss was about diet and exercise.

When I discovered the relationship between sleep and fat loss, I was actually pretty shocked. I could not believe that sleep had anything to do with my ability to lose weight, and it took a long time for me to process this information and really understand what occurs when you go to sleep at night and how it has anything to do with weight loss. Research published in *Annals of Internal Medicine* is one of many sources that establishes sleep as one of the most powerful elements to successful weight loss.

There simply isn't a diet pill on the planet that can mirror the benefits of sleep on weight loss as measured in this study, which compared two groups of overweight non-smokers on calorie-restricted diets for two weeks. One group got eight-and-a-half hours of sleep per night and the other slept only five-and-a-half hours per night.

Both groups had approximately 1,450 calories per day. After two weeks, the group that got more sleep lost 25% more fat than the ones who slept less. Surprisingly, participants burned more fat when as a result of getting more sleep!

Even more shocking, the ones who slept less lost 60% more muscle. Sleeping less caused the metabolism to shift and store fat at the expense of muscle. It was also revealed that the hormone levels in the ones who slept less had more of the hunger hormone ghrelin.

As if the reasons listed above were not enough to convince you to sleep longer, increased sleep has even more benefits! The metabolism is slowed down when we get less sleep and then the body starts to burn calories at a slower rate to preserve energy. In the study, people burned, on average, 400 more calories for sleeping three or more hours, which adds up to an additional 2,800 calories per week! When you get less sleep, however, the body tries to meet the energy requirements of longer waking hours by down shifting itself, which burns fewer calories and less fat. You can read the full study here: http://annals.org/aim/article/746184/insufficient-sleep-undermines-dietary-efforts-reduce-adiposity.

The bottom line is that if you want to burn fat, preserve muscle, and wake up less hungry, you need to focus on getting more sleep. Once you start getting good sleep, you will see how much more effective your weight-loss efforts will be.

FAT-BURNING ACTION #6: MOVE YOUR BODY

Despite popular opinion, it is absolutely possible to lose weight, and a ton of it, on this program without exercise. I'll say it again, **you do not have to exercise on this program and you will still lose fat**. In fact, in terms of getting the fastest results with your weight-loss efforts, it is much more efficient for you to eat foods that help your body rapidly burn fat than to eat bad foods and try to "burn it off" at the gym.

Some people say that weight loss is 80% diet and 20% exercise. That is wrong. Weight loss is 100% nutrition and exercise is an ancillary technique employed to build muscle, tone, shape, and sculpt your body.

Now don't get me wrong. I do believe exercise is very beneficial and there is definitely a time when it becomes necessary to incorporate into a healthy lifestyle. However, when you are just beginning a new lifestyle, I am a big believer in taking a gradual approach.

In the beginning of this program, there are so many internal metabolic changes occurring within your body and it is in full-on repair mode. It needs support in the form of superior nutrition, adequate hydration, and plentiful rest. During this healing process, it is best to reduce stress as much as possible and that includes physical exercise.

Walking, however, is part of The Perfect Day and I do not consider it "exercise" per se. Instead I call it "moving your body." With today's sedentary lifestyles and with most women having desk jobs, walking becomes a necessity to keep our body from becoming stiff, stale, and stagnant. Walking also helps with weight loss because it lowers stress and helps with circulation of nutrients throughout the body, which is necessary for optimal metabolism function. It also stimulates the fat-burning enzyme lipase. For this program, I suggest walking 20-30 minutes per day. Please note that this is optional and is not required, but is highly recommended.

If you are a fitness enthusiast and love to work out by doing other types of exercising, you can continue working out if you choose. If you choose to continue integrating rigorous exercise along with the 3X program, please just beware of your mindset. A problem I commonly see with women who exercise a lot is that they believe that working out entitles them to eat and drink whatever they want because they are still operating off the calories-in-versus-calories-out theory and that will absolutely keep you from getting the best results.

Let me tell you about Aimee. Aimee has been a personal trainer and a group exercise coach for over 20 years. She spent the last several years of her life trying to out-exercise a bad diet. Like many women, she felt that the three hours of exercise she did per day entitled her to eat whatever she wanted. But despite all of her efforts, she had 20 pounds that she just couldn't get rid of.

She realized while going through the 3X Program that she was seriously nutrient deficient and that no amount of exercise was going to get her body back to where she wanted it to be. Through the program, though, she got her nutrient levels back up and lost the 20 pounds just like that.

Thinking back to what you've learned thus far, have you been able to pinpoint the reason that Aimee initially was unable to lose weight? It was because despite exercising daily, she was only addressing the symptom (weight) without addressing the cause (nutritional deficiencies).

During phase 1, if you have more than 20 pounds to lose, and you want to exercise I ask that you only do light exercises such as walking, biking, swimming, or yoga. During the time when your body is healing and repairing, it can sometimes be counterproductive to overwhelm yourself with strenuous "boot camp" type exercising or hormone/stress elevating intense cardio. Those types of exercises put a lot of stress on your metabolism.

To further clarify, there's nothing wrong with having these stress factors on the body so long as the body is hormonally and nutritionally balanced on a cellular level. When it is, the body can easily handle these stress factors, as it is designed to do.

When the right messages are sent to the cells (in this case a nutritional reset, if you will), the body will say, "Oh, let's get rid of this fat. It shouldn't be here," and the body will just dump it— fast—without exercise. It can take a few weeks or a few months, depending on the amount of healing a person's body needs. But only after a person has reset their body on a cellular level (nutritionally) should one take up exercise.

So before you start to embark on heavy exercise, let's first get your metabolism optimized and your hormones balanced so that it feels safe in releasing fat. Once you are within a healthy weight range, exercise becomes very beneficial, as it is a necessary component to a healthy lifestyle.

The 3X Fitness Program begins in phase 2 after you have completed phase 1. Once most of the weight is gone and your metabolism is optimized, exercise is the next step to tone and sculpt your body (which can only be done through exercise).

FAT-BURNING ACTION #7: TRACKING YOUR PROGRESS

Study after study has proven that people who record their daily actions and track their progress lose more weight than those who don't, and in some cases even DOUBLE the amount lost versus those who don't. Wow! I can lose 2X more weight just simply by recording my daily actions? Sign me up!

Now let me be the first one to say that I used to think that journaling food was a total waste of time. In fact, it was my husband who first decided that we needed to do this. He created a checklist (those military men!) and listed out all the actions of The Perfect Day, printed it out, put it in a clipboard, and literally walked around with it all day writing things down and checking things off. I thought he was borderline nuts.

I couldn't believe he was so excited about this checklist! To him, it was everything and is what kept him moving forward on the program. Meanwhile, I couldn't for the life of me see how this little piece of paper could have any impact on my weight-loss results.

In the beginning, I actually tried to use it, but it would only last a day or two before I would forget to fill it out and began to think the whole thing was a little bit ridiculous. One day, after about a month of him using this checklist, I walked into his office and saw him pondering something. I asked him what he was doing, and he said that he realized that he stopped losing weight about a week ago and he was reviewing his daily checklists to find out what happened.

He started going through it in front of me and he realized that for the past week he hadn't gotten much sleep because of a big work project, and he also noted that he was drinking about ½ of the water that he was in the previous weeks. He got all giddy and said, "See, this is why I use a checklist. So that if something is off I can pinpoint exactly what happened and then remedy it." I was in utter shock and had the biggest realization of my weight-loss life. Instead of guessing what happened or chalking it up to saying the program stopped working and jumping off to start the next new diet fad, just like that he had debugged his weight-loss plateau and knew exactly what to do to keep moving forward and start getting results again.

I realized at that moment the value of tracking daily actions. Instead of viewing it as something that was tedious or unnecessary, I shifted my viewpoint and saw it as an effective tool that was going to assist me in reaching my goal. I learned that the power of this tool was that by recording my daily actions and tracking my progress,

I would be able to identify the things that were blocking me from success. So I began recording everything and experienced firsthand how much it actually effected my motivation and consistency with sticking to the plan.

Another thing I love about tracking is how much better I do on the program when recording my daily actions. It helped me reach my goal weight so much faster because I was able to identify old habits that I might have never even noticed because I was so used to doing them. But since I knew that I was going to record it, I didn't want to do anything bad because I didn't want to have to write that down. This helped me so much if I was ever having a weak moment. I just simply thought about how I would feel about myself when I had to write down having that piece of cake or slice of pizza. I didn't want to write it down, so therefore I didn't end up having it. Can you see how powerful this tool is in keeping you on track? It's amazing!

Since then I've become a die-hard advocate of recording daily actions and tracking progress. To aid the process, I created the 3X Weight Loss Progress Tracker mobile app. It allows you set up a fit profile to track your progress, a daily checklist to track your perfect days, a nutrition diary to log your meals, and even a way to participate in challenges and rewards to keep you motivated. You can also get support from other participants and gain access to a wide variety of tools to make active, healthy living easier and more fun. It truly does make all the difference in staying motivated and consistent.

Using the 3X Weight Loss Progress Tracker App is the key to implementing The Perfect Day into your life so that it becomes part of your normal routine. If followed consistently, you will establish a daily routine that keeps your body in fat-burning mode 24/7.

You can start your free trial of the 3X Weight Loss Program, which includes the progress tracker app, at www.3xweightloss.com/free-trial.

WHY IS THE PERFECT DAY IMPORTANT?

It wasn't until I fully implemented The Perfect Day and did it consistently enough to develop new habits that I no longer thought about it as a diet. It was a healthy lifestyle that I was working towards perfecting, and every day and week it got easier and I got closer and closer to my goal. I became more efficient with the way that I did things, how I shopped for food, and how I prepped my food. When I went out to restaurants, I knew exactly what to order. If I ever went astray from the plan and had a bad day, it didn't turn into a bad week, or a bad month, or a bad year. There was no "crashing and burning." There was no more searching, hoping, and praying that I would find a better way. I didn't have to obsess anymore. I just knew exactly what to do to get re-focused and back on track.

With The Perfect Day, I've made it easy for you to implement a daily fat-burning routine so that you naturally reset your metabolism, balance your hormones, and reach optimal levels of health.

THE KEY TO RAPID FAT LOSS IS TO FOLLOW THE PERFECT DAY. It is the number of perfect days you have that determines the speed at which you lose weight.

The 3X Perfect Day has been tested and proven to produce three times faster results than just dieting on your own and is WHY the program is called 3X Weight Loss.

The more perfect days you follow, the closer and closer you're going to get towards your weight-loss goal.

Conversely, the fewer perfect days you have, the slower you're going to reach your weight-loss goal. It is up to you how quickly you want to do this. You can, however, do this program at your own pace. This is a lifestyle, not a race. Implementing any one of these daily fat-burning actions will completely change the way your metabolism performs.

For women who are ready to go all in and get the best results possible, I recommend implementing each of the daily fat-burning actions into your life. If you aren't ready to go full force, then you can simply focus on adding in one action every day until you have it mastered and then move onto the next action and so forth until you have them all implemented into a normal daily routine.

The truth is you are just a number of Perfect Days away from having the body you want.

With that said, I have created The Perfect Day Manifesto to remind you daily of the purpose of doing Perfect Days.

The secret to getting fast results and reaching your goal, whether its ten pounds or 100 pounds, is to **follow The Perfect Day every day**. Again, the more perfect days you have, the faster you will reach your goal!

THE PERFECT DAY
MANIFESTO

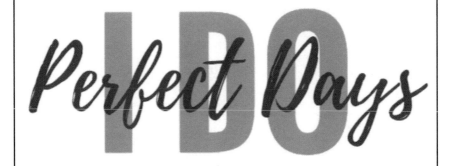

I MAKE
MY DAY
I DECIDE
MY ACTIONS

I CONTROL
MY CHOICES

I CREATE
MY BODY

I CHOOSE
MY HEALTH

I AM JUST A PERFECT DAY AWAY!

ROUTINES

Now that you know the seven daily fat-burning actions that make up The Perfect Day and exactly what to do daily to get healthy and reach your goal weight, let's talk about routines. According to Oxford dictionary, the definition of routine is "a sequence of actions regularly followed; a fixed program." Simply put, the things you do on a daily basis make up your routine.

"But Laura, you don't understand! I have a full-time job! I have four kids! I volunteer at my church! I don't have time to grocery shop! I don't have time to juice vegetables! I can't possibly pack my meals a head of time! There's no way I can do this!" I can already hear the excuses and so I'm going to be frank with you: Your current routine is what created your current body. If you want to change your body you have to change your routine. Having no time, being stressed out, and constantly running around like a chicken with your head cut off has gotten you into the situation you are currently in. And it's likely a miserable place to be. I know because I was there. And it wasn't until I realized that if I ever wanted to be happy with my body, I needed to quit using the "no time" excuse and make my health a priority.

How do you make time? You plan, get organized, and become efficient. Doesn't sound fun, I know. But I promise your life will never be the same (in a good way) once you master the skills I'm going to teach you in the next section.

The truth is that your daily routine is either helping you lose weight or it's making you fat. Either it's contributing to your health, or its taking years away from your life. This may sound harsh, but it is absolutely the way it works.

Before starting this program, you need to ask yourself if you're willing to make the necessary adjustments to your current routine so that you can establish a healthy lifestyle that will get you the body you desire. Do you want to change your routine from one that is damaging to your health and storing fat to one that will bring you toward optimum health while melting fat off your body 24/7? I hope you answered YES to that question! If you did, then keep reading!

I've given you all the information you need and shown you the exact steps of what to do. But now you're probably wondering, *how* do you do it? How do you implement the things I've laid out for you and make them a part of your normal, everyday routine?

By doing the seven daily fat-burning actions of The Perfect Day consistently until they become a new routine.

Remember, the definition of routine is "a sequence of actions regularly followed; a fixed program." Once you get the hang of The Perfect Day and do it for a minimum of 30 days, it will become a normal routine, and you'll thank me for helping to make your life so much more simple and effective, I promise. So if you're ready, join me in the next chapter and let's get this party started!

CHAPTER 7

GOALS, MOTIVATION, SELF-DISCIPLINE, WILLPOWER, AND CONSISTENCY

A lot of women think that the reason they can't stick to a plan long enough to reach their goal is because they aren't motivated or they don't have enough willpower. They say things like, "I can't seem to stay away from bad foods," or "I'm not motivated enough to go to the gym." Does this sound familiar? If you are one of these women, I'm here to tell you that none of these things are true. And luckily for you, on this program they will not be of concern.

When you aren't hungry, don't have cravings, and aren't required to go to the gym every day to get results, who needs willpower? And when you're actually seeing the scale drop a pound or more each day, inches melt right off your body, and you feel better than you have in years, who needs more motivation than that?

Willpower and motivation are a thing of the past! These are for people who are dieting by starving and suffering with exhausting fitness programs day in and day out (and are still not seeing results). When you give your body what it needs, like you will on this program, you will experience a whole new realm of self-discipline like you've never thought possible. And you'll discover that it's been inside you this whole time. You didn't have to do anything to get it other than give your body what it needs. Weird how that works, huh? So let's talk about this thing called self-discipline.

In case you've labeled yourself as someone who "doesn't have self-discipline," I want you to know that no one was born with more self-discipline than you. Self-discipline is not genetic. It's not something that grows on trees. It's actually created a single step at a time.

Self-discipline:

- Is the *result* of doing what you say you will do
- Is something that has to be exercised as it doesn't just happen over night
- Comes from consistently doing actions that are in alignment with your goals and not doing actions that are not in alignment with your goals

It is really that simple.

Not surprisingly, self-discipline and goal achievement go hand in hand. So before we discuss how to get self-discipline, let's talk about goals.

WHAT IS A GOAL?

Let's first start by defining what a goal is. Goal achievement is about these three things:

1. Intention: A strong sense of knowing what you want and intending on getting it.
2. Planning: Taking the time necessary to create a plan and then getting organized and preparing to set yourself up for success.
3. Taking action: DOING the actions of your plan every day.

To most people, goals are more like dreams. They are things they wish for in their mind and think about wanting to achieve but never actually do. The concept of goals and dreams are often confused. But the difference between a goal and a dream is that dream is something you think about and wish somehow happens for you someday. A goal is something you set out to achieve and then have to DO actions in the real world that will bring you towards that goal. NOTE: A goal can be a dream as well, but you need to take action to achieve your goals, not just dream about them.

We all know how easy it is to set goals, but achieving them can be a whole different beast. There are way too many distractions in our everyday life that act as barriers for reaching our goals. Be it your demanding career, maintaining a household, or taking care of your family and all of their needs, there are always going to be things that suddenly pop up and try to take you off the path of reaching your goals. Which is why if you're not 100% dedicated and committed to your goal with a solid plan in place, there will be a million other things that come up and give you all the reasons and excuses you need not to do it. In turn, you'll be unhappy and hopeless about changing your health and your body.

You must stay focused on the target and make a healthy lifestyle a priority!

Now, I completely understand that this is easier said than done. However, by having a plan in place that guides you every step of the way and keeps you on track no matter what, reaching your goal will become an actuality and not just a dream never to be attained.

DISCIPLINE EQUALS FREEDOM

I actually used to hate the concept of being disciplined. Even the word discipline used to scare me. It was probably because while I was growing up, my father prided himself on being a disciplinarian.

His way of parenting was all about following the rules, punishment, and consequences. As someone who has always been a "free spirit," I had a lot of resentment around discipline because of that extreme structure growing up. Let's just say I was grounded a lot!

Surprisingly, even though I despised discipline, structure, and the like, I ended up falling in love and marrying a man who was formerly in the military. Not only was he formerly in the military, but he was in the US Navy Special Operations, Explosive Ordinance Disposal. In other words, he diffused bombs. While he was in the military, his life literally depended upon following very precise procedures. Every day he had to adhere to very strict discipline, follow standard operating procedures, and ensure he got results by following protocols. It became ingrained in him and became a part of who he is.

Even though we're two totally different personalities, we love each other so deeply. And shockingly enough, one of the things that I love most my husband is the fact that he does have a lot of structure; it benefits our family and relationship in a really great way.

It's so funny because when I cook something, I tend to just toss random ingredients together, never measure anything, and pop it in the oven until it looks done. And I absolutely never follow recipes exactly by the book. My husband, on the other hand, is the complete opposite.

The second he starts the grill, he puts his timer on. He knows exactly how many minutes to keep something on and how much seasoning to use. He is very precise, logical, and calculated. Everything is about checklists, formulas, procedures, etc. I must admit, though, his military training around discipline and structure has served him very well in life both personally and professionally.

So it was through our relationship that I actually got to see for the first time that discipline was not a bad thing. And I learned that in order to live a successful life, some level of discipline was needed.

My perspective on discipline further shifted after becoming familiar with the concept "discipline equals freedom." Jocko Willink, a former Navy SEAL, coined the phrase and my husband introduced it to me. What it means is that you have to be disciplined in order to have freedom. Everyone wants freedom, right? Well you can only have it if you can be disciplined enough to get it. In his book *Extreme Ownership*, Jocko explains how being disciplined as a Navy SEAL allowed him to be more efficient, perform at higher levels, and create more time.

The following is an excerpt from *Extreme Ownership* on the principle that discipline equals freedom.

I learned in the SEAL training that if I wanted any extra time to study the academic material we were given, prepare our room and my uniforms for an inspection, or just stretch out aching muscles, I had to make that time because it did not exist on the written schedule. When I checked into my first SEAL team, that practice continued. If I wanted extra time to work on my gear, clean my weapons, study tactics or new technology, I needed to make that time. The only way you could make time was to get up early. That took discipline.

Waking up early was the first example I noticed in the SEAL teams in which discipline was really the difference between being good and being exceptional. I saw it with some of the older, experienced SEALs. Those who were at work before everyone else were the ones who were considered the best "operators." That meant they had the best field craft, the most squared away gear, they were the best shots, and they were the most respected. It all tied into discipline. By discipline, I mean an intrinsic self-discipline – a matter of personal will. The best SEALs I worked with were invariably the most disciplined. They woke up early. They worked out every day.

They studied tactics and technology. They practiced their craft. Some of them even went out on the town, drank, and stayed out until the early hours of the morning. But they still woke up early and maintained discipline at every level.

The temptation to take the easy road is always there. It is as easy as staying in bed in the morning and sleeping in. But discipline is paramount to ultimate success and victory from any leader and any team.

After reading this book and learning more about the concept, for the first time I truly understood how being disciplined enough to live a healthy life actually does give me freedom and creates more time.

Freedom from what? Just fill in the blank. For me it was freedom from hating how I looked when I saw myself in the mirror. Freedom from negative self-talk. Freedom from not feeling and looking my best. Freedom from food addictions and cravings. Freedom from obsessing over my body. Freedom from dieting and exercising. The list goes on and on. As a result, because I had enough self-discipline to follow the plan and do perfect days consistently enough until they became habits, I can honestly say that I now have total body freedom.

Many women have told me that the reason that they can't lose weight is because they don't have time. Trust me, if anyone understands this scenario, it's me. I have two kids, two dogs, a husband, a career, and a household to run. On top of that, I live 30 minutes from my son's school, so I spend two hours a day just driving him to and from school. I totally get it: We are all very busy. We live hectic, stressful lives and between our careers, family, and home life, there simply aren't enough hours in the day.

Because of life's pressures and demands, your health is one of the first things that gets deprioritized and is put on the back burner. Unfortunately, as a result of this deprioritization, many other areas in your life will suffer as well. After years of doing this, you may wake up one day and be 30 or more pounds overweight, have aches and pains, and don't feel as good as you once did. Now you're on a downward spiral and it becomes a slippery slope that just keeps getting worse and worse.

So it is *critical* that you adapt the mindset of discipline equals freedom and create systems in your life that foster increased productivity. This leads to more free time, less stress, and more freedom.

Once you can get into the frame of mind that discipline is not necessarily a bad thing, you'll be on the fast track towards success. By setting up structure inside your life, making a plan, sticking to it, and following it, you will eventually have more time and freedom from all of those negative aspects that come from being overweight.

Having now shed light on how helpful and important discipline is in losing weight, I hope that you're excited about the structure you'll have that will facilitate reaching your weight-loss goal!

LET'S GET STARTED!

Here is the three-step formula for self-discipline:

1. First, you must determine a clearly defined goal. Example: I want to lose 20 pounds so that I can feel good about myself, have more energy, increase my self-confidence, and go to the pool with my kids without worrying about my body.
2. Next, you need to list out the actionable steps that if taken, will achieve that goal. I've already done this for you with The Perfect Day.

3.   Lastly, do those steps consistently to see results and repeat every single day until the full goal is achieved.

That's all self-discipline is, and doing the three steps above will result in you having it. It's not a complex thing. When weight loss is done correctly and done according to the way your body naturally functions, it is actually a very simple process. Stop doing the things that hinder it and start doing things that nourish it. Do these specific things every day and sooner than you know it, you're going to be at your goal weight. Now, let's further break down these steps so that you fully understand each one.

STEP 1: DETERMINE YOUR GOAL

What is it that you want? Do you want to lose 30 pounds or 50 pounds? Why? Is it so that you can look better, feel better, have better health, live longer for your children and grandchildren, pay less insurance cost, get a better job? Whatever the reason for wanting to lose weight, write that down. Example: "I want to lose 30 pounds so that I can have more energy and better health to be a better mom for my kids and a sexier wife for my husband." Be specific. Whatever it is, write it down on a piece of paper **right now**.

No goal is too big, too small, or too ridiculous. But you must actually write it down or type it up. Don't just say, I know my goal, it is in my head. There are a lot of random things in your head, and you need to make an assertion—a statement—that this is not just another random thought floating through your mind; this is a declaration of something you are going to achieve in the real world. You are not going to achieve this goal in dreamland, so quit thinking about it and write it down on paper in the real world.

Identify your long-term goal, which would be the total amount of weight you want to lose, but then I want you to take it a step further and break that goal into smaller goals. I suggest setting 30-day goals that you can focus on hitting one month at a time. For example, if you want to lose a total of 100 pounds, it might feel overwhelming at first, but if you break this goal up into 30-day chunks and only focus on that 30-day goal, it will become a lot more achievable.

On the 3X Weight Loss Program, the average weight loss that can be experienced in 30 days is 15 pounds. However, I have had people lose a lot more than that; it just depends how well you follow The Perfect Day. So let's say that you have 100 pounds to lose and you break that up into several 30-day goals. Your first goal is to just lose 15 pounds in the first 30 days. Set that goal and keep yourself focused on reaching that one goal by following the rest of the goal formula below. Adjust this scenario based on the amount of weight that you want to lose, and you will have an estimate of how long it should take you and it will give you your target for each 30 days of the entire cycle of reaching the total goal.

Ok, so you have your goals written down right? The next step is creating a plan.

STEP 2: CREATE A PLAN

What you need to know about goal attainment is that to make the decision once to lose weight, when you initially write your goal down, is not sufficient to get you the results you want. In order for weight loss to work for you, you have to make certain decisions anew *every day*. Then and only then will you start to see the results that you set out to get. So remember, this is not just a one-time decision you are making to "go on a diet."

Chances are, it took you several years to gain the weight, but the good news is that it only takes a few weeks or months to lose it. Nevertheless, it is an ongoing decision that you have to make every day.

Part A

Step two of the formula is two-fold. Part A is to create a plan. An example of a plan would be to follow the 3X Weight Loss Protocol. It includes setting aside time to plan your meals for the week, shopping for them, and preparing them ahead of time so that you have them readily available when you are hungry. A plan would also include how you are going to get the support and accountability you may need while reaching your goal weight.

Unfortunately, most women try to "wing it" when they go on a diet and one of the biggest reasons for diet failure is not being prepared and lack of support. I can't stress enough how important following a plan of action is.

Part B

The second part of the plan is to take your overall plan and break it into steps, which are the daily actions that need to be done each day to take you from where you are right now to achieving your goal.

For instance, eating healthy meals for breakfast, lunch, dinner, and snacks would be considered the daily actions. Going on a walk, joining a support group forum, and talking to other women about your challenges and successes would be daily actions.

Avoiding temptations or foods that are going to set you back would also be daily actions.

STEP 3: TAKE ACTION

A plan with these things needs to be not only planned for, but also DONE.

Step three is as simple as that! DO the daily actions repeatedly until you reach your weight-loss goal.

CONTRIBUTING ACTIONS VS. SUBTRACTING ACTIONS

The specific daily actions that are going to take you from where you are right now to achieving your goals are called contributing actions. These are the daily, fat-burning actions that make up The Perfect Day. There are also subtracting actions, which are actions that move you further away from your goal. As bold as it may sound, subtracting actions are the actions that have given you the body you currently have. It is now time to focus ONLY on doing as many contributing actions as you can each day!

You have the choice every day either to do contributing actions (actions that contribute to your health goals) or subtracting actions (actions that take you away from your health goals). As a reminder, contributing actions are the steps of The Perfect Day, and the actions you want to take to reach your health and weight-loss goals.

To keep it really simple, here is how you can view this. You only have these two choices at all times: contributing actions or subtracting actions.

- ☐ In regard to your health: get better or get worse.
- ☐ In regard to weight loss; lose weight or gain weight.
- ☐ In regard to food choices: burn fat or store fat.

THE BIGGEST SECRET TO HAVING SELF-DISCIPLINE

It's really simple: A disciplined person simply does a high number of contributing actions on a daily basis and does not do subtracting actions. All discipline is, when you break it down, is having a clearly defined goal, working out the actions necessary to achieve that goal, and doing those actions every single day until that goal is achieved.

It's not a complex willpower, mental thing that you have to go through.

All you have to do is know the steps that are going to take you to your goal and do them consistently. DO the steps every day, that's all you have to do!

It is really not any more complicated or difficult than that, ladies. But notice, I did say *consistently*. You have to do these contributing actions every day if you really want to reach your goal weight, not just a few times a week.

By implementing The Perfect Day and by keeping track of your contributing actions each day, you will gain more momentum and lose more weight. This automatically increases your motivation because you start to SEE the rewards of your efforts.

WEIGHT-LOSS MOMENTUM

Ever wonder why one little indulgence can slow down or even reverse your weight-loss progress? It's because of a concept called weight-loss momentum. Since you now know how your body burns fat and how it stores it, now is a good time to let you know that cheating on the plan can set you back three to five days. If you decide to go out Friday night and "celebrate" the fact that you've lost seven pounds in a week, you won't actually end up burning fat again until maybe Monday or Tuesday of the next week. If you end up doing that just a couple of times in a row, you are going to find that a few months have gone by and you only ended up losing seven pounds of the 37 that you really wanted to lose. It is just not worth it.

Once you get into fat-burning mode, YOU WANT TO STAY THERE until you reach your goal as this is the EASIEST WAY to reach your goal. Otherwise, you are adding weeks, months, and even years to reaching your target weight by confusing your body back and forth between fat-burning mode and fat-storing mode.

This is the trap that most women are in and have been in for years. It is the reason women feel they can never have a perfect body. So don't short yourself by staying disciplined for a few days, cheating, getting back on, and then cheating again. Go all out! Bang it out! Reach your goal and go enjoy your life. What is the point of spending your entire life struggling to reach your optimum weight and health?

Don't you want to be there now and live out the rest of your life with the benefits of being leaner and healthier? Well then it is time to be honest with yourself. Doing the things you've done in the past hasn't gotten you anywhere.

Everyone wants to lose weight, have a perfect body, and better health. But it simply isn't as easy as taking a magic pill, using a body wrap, or rubbing some lotion on your skin. Real health and long-lasting weight loss requires lifestyle changes. If you are not willing to make a healthy lifestyle a priority, then you are not ready to lose weight.

Remember, discipline equals freedom. If you stay disciplined and follow the program you will be FREE of all the excess weight that is holding you back.

You bought this book and are still reading, so I know deep down you are ready for a real lifestyle change and that you just needed to find the right plan that would truly get you to your goal weight. And THAT is exactly what I have provided you with. So please, take what you learn in this book and APPLY it. You'll be experiencing quite a bit of change as you do though, so in the next chapter, I will detail what to expect while on the program.

CHAPTER 8

WHAT TO EXPECT

The average person who embarks on the 3X journey loses 26.7 pounds in 60 days. Nope, no typo there. 26.7! After the first two months, clients generally lose ten to fifteen pounds per month, but it wholly depends on the person and these results are not guaranteed. Just like anything else, you are only going to get out of the program what you put into it.

No other weight-loss program that I know of has achieved what 3X has in terms of these kinds of results. And the benefits of this program go way beyond just weight loss. Here are exact words from women who are currently on the program and the benefits they've realized.

"More energy, better sleep."

"Handled my high blood pressure, insomnia, tummy aches & headaches Knowledge about nutrition."

"My skin was smoother, no heartburn, no gas or cramping. Normal bowel movements (I know, gross, but very noticeable difference)."

"Happier."

"It becomes a habit of eating cleaner (healthy)."

"My blood pressure is now normal. I have no more digestion issues. I feel happier. All around is a better way of life for me. I'm still not perfect. But it doesn't have to be. But it is right. That's what matters."

"Considerably regulated my cycle. No more iron deficiency anemia."

"My family eats better."

"More energy, much less gas and bloating, better sleep and clearer skin

"My children have lost 35 pounds combined!"

"Education. Support. Energy. Clearer skin. Regularly going to the bathroom. No acid reflux."

"Better sleep, total elimination of night sweats (more like night drenching) more consistent energy levels, flatter tummy, the excitement and joy that comes from being in control of my body."

"So much knowledge about food! We out less, eat together more and eat so much better, focusing on making nutrients taste good! Clearer skin and more energy!"

"More energy, and ability to focus and my skin rashes are going away."

"No more snoring. Hardly any gas. Sleep apnea is not as frequent"

"Clearer skin, less inflammation (I have psoriatic arthritis), better sleep, better energy, no acid reflux, lost 32 pounds and a lot fewer cravings for sweets."

"More energy, better image of myself."

"No more heartburn, bloating, constipation; increased energy, decreased depression and anxiety."

"No more stress, high blood pressure, pre-diabetes or arthritis aches and pains."

"More sleep, energy, clarity and focus."

"More mental clarity, fewer headaches. More in control of my weight, which has brought more happiness!"

"I have noticed much-improved sleep and overall wellbeing"

"Healthier hair, skin, and nails for sure!"

"Feel better overall—hard to put my finger on it—definitely fewer pains and body problems than I had before, more energy, etc. You probably want specific points but it's hard to pinpoint! Just a big difference lol. My life and joy no longer revolve around food as it once did, which is a big deal. The addiction gets broken."

"My husband and I were able to go on hikes this week with a hiking group...something we would not have been in shape for two months ago."

"I felt really good and with no acid reflux and inflammation which caused me joint pain."

See what I mean?! This is exciting because you are about to begin implementing everything that you've learned so far and set yourself on the path to rapid fat burning, so I'm *super* excited for you. So I hope you are ready to dive in and give it your all so that you can experience these types of results as well. Now we'll move on to how to get the most success out of this program.

TIPS FOR SUCCESS

I've nicknamed the first week of the program "Hell Week." I know that sounds scary, but it's not. It's called Hell Week because for the first week it might seem a little challenging, but this is only because you are switching it up, changing old routines, getting rid of bad habits, and establishing new routines. It can all seem pretty overwhelming at first, but just bear with it for the first week.

If you stay the course and follow The Perfect Day every day your first week and do the best you can, you'll get through this week with no problem. And the good news is that you'll almost immediately begin seeing results and that's what's going to give you the motivation to get you through.

Here's what to expect: Week one you might be a little cranky. Week two you will be doing the weight-loss happy dance, promise. Don't worry, once you've broken the sugar addictions and the bad food habits, the program will seem effortless and actually becomes a normal part of your everyday life.

Let's talk about that sugar addiction for a moment. Breaking the cravings for sugar and junk food can make you not feel good and you will likely experience some withdrawal symptoms. Some people do not have any withdrawal symptoms and others feel crappy for just a few days; it all depends on each person. So please be prepared should you go through withdrawal or detox symptoms.

As you embark on this program, the single most important piece of advice that would give you the best chance of success is to be prepared with weekly meal prep. This is absolutely the simplest way to stick to the program and reach your weight-loss goals. It may seem at first that you are spending a lot of time meal prepping, but once you get the hang of it, it becomes a weekly ritual that cuts out several hours per week in the kitchen and saves you hundreds of dollars on food each month.

In the next section, I will cover meal prepping. It includes a step-by-step meal prepping system that walks you through exactly how and what to prepare to get the most success out of this program.

Another tip is to keep everything as simple as possible so that you don't overwhelm yourself. This is why I created The Perfect Day: for simplicity. There's no reason to try a new recipe for every meal for every day (though you can). I suggest keeping it simple because that's what's going to be easiest for you until you get used to your new routine. So start by just following The Perfect Day and do it daily until you feel confident and comfortable enough to move on to new recipes.

NO CHEATING!

Not on Fridays. Not on Saturdays. Not once every two weeks. Don't cheat at all. Cheating is going to set you back three or so days each time. That starts to add up, and you don't want to short yourself the success that is possible with this program.

The good news is that once your body gets in fat-burning mode, you're actually burning fat pretty much 24/7 because there's really no other choice for your body; there's nothing else in there to burn. Your body runs off glucose and if you aren't getting it from sugar or other bad carbs, then it's going to get its energy from your stored fat cells, which is what you want.

So it gets really exciting because it's one of those things that once you get into fat-burning mode, you just keep going and going and going and you don't want to interrupt that process by cheating.

So no cheating, ladies! You've had the past however many years to eat as many bad foods as you wanted to. It's time to buckle down and do this all out for the next few weeks (or for however long it takes for you to reach your weight-loss goal).

I created something called a cheat card to read so that you can be mindful of the choices you are making and the consequences. So read this before you decide to cheat and I bet if you read this before deciding to cheat you might just change your mind!

WAIT!!!

BEFORE YOU CHEAT READ THIS:

 I am aware that the food I am about to eat will develop into new fat cells around my belly, hips and thighs.

 I am OK with gaining 1-2 pounds from eating these foods.

 I understand that by eating these foods I will not burn fat for up to 3 days.

 I realize that by eating these foods I will be creating more bad habits, food addicitons and sugar cravings.

 I understand that eating bad foods can create nutritional deficiencies that will slow my metabolism.

 I understand that sugar feeds cancer and breeds bad bacteria and yeast that can take over my digestive system making it nearly impossible for me to lose weight and get the body I want.

DO I REALLY WANT TO DO THIS?

Now, as much as I recommend NOT cheating, I also know that we are human. So don't beat yourself up if you have a bad day or even a bad week. The most incredible thing about this program is the fact that all you have to do is jump right back on the Perfect Day and you will start to lose weight again quickly. So again, this is another reason why the Perfect Day is your blueprint for life.

Lastly, if you want to get the most out of this program and really ensure you get great results, I highly recommend becoming a member of 3X Weight Loss and going through the video coaching program for more in-depth training as well as gaining access to hundreds of recipes, the support group, and the additional tools and resources.

You can begin your success story with a free trial of 3X Weight Loss at www.3xweightloss.com/free-trial.

Audrey Pi-Gonzalez Lost 75 Pounds in just 4 Months!

> *Every year on my birthday I'd tell myself I needed to do something about my weight, but I didn't know how or where to start. 15 years passed before I became successful in losing weight.*

> *Last year, in 2016, I tried Weight Watchers and did the whole counting points thing. This was exhausting, and I felt I was spending way too much time scanning labels at the store. I did lose 25lbs but managed to gain 10 of them back. I told myself this is the year I will not lie to myself on my birthday in September. I started the 3X Weight Loss Program on May 15, 2017 and at the time wore a size 26 and in some clothes a 28.*

> *This year when my birthday came, I had lost 75 lbs. That's right, 75lbs from May 15, 2017 to September 15, 2017. I'm now a size 18 that's 4 pants sizes!!! Of course, I had to get all new clothes; darn—I know.*

In these three months, I haven't deviated from the program once. There are no cheat days. No cheat meals. The cravings stopped long ago.

I still have more weight to lose but this program has provided me with the knowledge to make the right choice for my health and me. This program has changed my life for the better and can't thank Laura Sales enough for sharing all her knowledge.

I no longer dread sitting in a booth, wondering if the airplane seat belt would fit, or feel other people watch as the big girl walks down the street or in a store.

This is a life-changing program what I fully endorse and encourage other women to participate in. -Audrey Pi Gonzalez

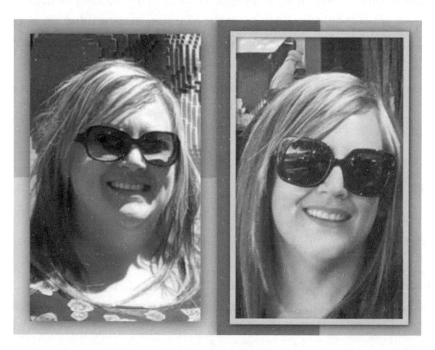

SECTION 3

MAKING 3X WEIGHT LOSS WORK FOR YOU

The 3X Weight Loss Program is a definite lifestyle adjustment for most women, especially for those who are accustomed to eating conventional foods, like processed bread, chips, cookies, crackers, frozen dinners, and canned foods—but that doesn't mean it has to be hard! After all, the harder something is, the less likely you are to stick to it, and that would defeat the purpose of the whole program.

Since 3X has become a way of life for my family and me, I have learned through trial and error how to weave the program's principals seamlessly into my life and I want to share what I've learned with you. In this last section, I'm going to give you as many lifestyle tips as possible so you can make the program even more doable. You will have no excuses to get started on your new healthy lifestyle program!

CHAPTER 9

THE RESPONSIBILITY OF SELF-CARE

When I became a wife and a mother, I soon realized that life was no longer just about me. My role as a woman now that I was a mom and a wife meant that I was responsible for caring for my family, and that also meant caring for their health. That last part was something I had never thought about before.

Prior to developing this program, I just thought that being healthy was a matter of genes or good luck. It wasn't until I took matters into my own hands that I understood that good health is something you are rewarded with IF you are proactive and take good care of yourself. It then dawned on me that I now had a massive responsibility and that I needed to do whatever it took to truly take care of my family by ensuring they are healthy *no matter what*.

At first, I was overwhelmed and wasn't sure I wanted to handle that amount of responsibility. I had no idea where to start. I was never taught how to be healthy in high school or college and I didn't learn it from my parents as they were always so busy working to put food on the table. I had to learn all of this through my own experience in becoming a wife. And it was quite a learning curve

167

because up until getting married, I had rarely ever cooked and the microwave had been my best friend! The fact of the matter was that if I wasn't nuking something I would just eat out because it was just so convenient. I soon learned that convenience also comes with serious health consequences.

When I faced the harsh reality that it was my responsibility that my family ate healthy, I then began to view it as a privilege and my duty. How amazing to be knowledgeable about what my family needs, not to get the bare minimum to survive, but to actually thrive and be the healthiest they can! To honor this, I set aside time to plan out the weekly meals and to go grocery shopping for the best-quality food that I can find. And let me be clear: I still don't love to cook but I do it because I know it's the best thing for our health.

Many women don't make this commitment to themselves (or their family) of putting their health first. Instead, they opt for convenience and end up doing whatever is cheapest or quickest. They use the excuse that they don't have time or can't afford to eat healthy but the truth is, they simply don't plan ahead.

I realize that not everyone reading this book has other people to care for, but regardless of your situation, it's important to acknowledge how critical self-care over convenience is. If you really want to get healthy and lose weight, you have to change your mindset and accept that you and your family are worth it. Whatever activities you are doing that are keeping you from "having time" need to be re-prioritized.

To close out the chapter, here's a letter I received from my client Elainna C. She shares her experiences as a mom attempting to properly care for and nourish herself and her family and the benefits they all realized after embarking on the 3X journey.

A few months ago, I got sick and tired of being overweight. I realized that I always felt tired, wiped out, and exhausted.

For me, this is what "normal" felt like. As a mom of three beautiful girls, who is quickly approaching 40, I thought to myself, "Wow, so this is what being almost 40 feels like?" Ugh...I honestly felt like I had aged 10 years in the past five years, and I did not like it one bit.

Like millions of mothers (and dads putting on sympathy weight) my age, I seemed to put on 10 pounds per child, or so I thought. At the age of 31, one year after giving birth to my third daughter, I had lost all of my baby weight. But, within 12 months, I found the 15 pounds that I lost, and they decided to park themselves on my hips for the next seven years. In fact, no matter how much I dieted or exercised the pounds kept finding me. I could run, but I couldn't hide!

While I don't consider myself obese by any measure, it's been about eight years since I wore a size four or six, and I was growing tired of being self-conscious about my pant size. I knew I was facing an uphill battle if I didn't buckle down and get my act together.

Being overweight, I felt crappy more often than I'd like to admit. But, I wasn't attributing my discomfort to what it said on the scale, I was attributing it to stress, working full-time, and approaching 40. As a former skinny girl who was horrified by her reflection in the mirror, I decided I had to lose weight. At the time, I was more motivated by wearing a size four again than I was by getting healthy. Why? Because I was under the impression that I was relatively healthy already... and boy was I wrong. Dead wrong.

When I was a stay-at-home mom, I ate much healthier, but as I began working 40, 50, and 60-hour workweeks, it was all at the expense of my family's health. Before I knew it, 90 percent of what we ate came from a box or a can; we ate very little fresh food!

My freezer was packed full of frozen dinners. I ate wheat bread, pasta, and tortillas and I ate out at least once a week. As a busy working mom, I bought "convenience foods." I cooked less and used the microwave more. If I had a choice between a salad and a frozen dinner, I'd opt for the frozen dinner in a heartbeat and I'm sure many parents can relate. I justified my choices by thinking, "I work full-time, I'm doing the best that I can do."

Before switching from processed foods to wholesome foods, I was one of those people who laughed at the idea of spending more money on healthier food. I knew I should've been eating healthier than I was, but I explained away my unhealthy choices by convincing myself that it was okay to eat processed food because I was just too busy to do anything else.

When I began 3X Weight Loss, something magical happened. I started to feel different. My headaches disappeared, my knees stopped hurting, my energy came back, and my brain fog was gone. I didn't attribute these changes to losing weight. I realized they had to do with what I was putting in my body. Suddenly, I began to see processed foods very differently.

When I decided to start 3X, I never thought twice about how it would affect my family. I knew I could continue buying them junk while buying healthy food for me, but after getting educated on the health benefits of eating clean, I didn't want to keep feeding my family processed foods, such as frozen dinners, packaged crackers, canned soups, ranch dressings loaded with MSG, fruit snacks and the like to my family.

On about day ten of 3X Weight Loss, my 14-year-old daughter runs into my home office while I'm writing and squeals, "Mom, I lost five pounds!" On about day 14, I walk into the bathroom as my 13-year-old daughter is getting ready in front of the mirror, and suddenly, I realize that she too is looking leaner and healthier than she did before I embarked on my weight-loss journey. I found my daughters' weight loss amusing, because I never intended that to happen.

If my kids were at their ideal body weight, I wouldn't be writing about them losing a few pounds, but like millions of American children, they had "room for improvement" in the health department. So, our entire household has benefited by my mission to switch to a healthier lifestyle, and I know that just about all children in the United States would be healthier if their parents ditched the white flour, sugar, and highly processed foods for wholesome, one-ingredient foods, such as meat, fruits and vegetables, nuts and seeds.

Even if parents shudder in fear, "My kids will never eat like that," it's not up to the kids. Parents need to be parents, don't they? Cheeseballs or a salad? Parents, you make the choice when you go to the store and plop down the money. If junk food is not available in the house, your kids aren't going to eat it. If your child is struggling with their weight, you have to make an executive decision.

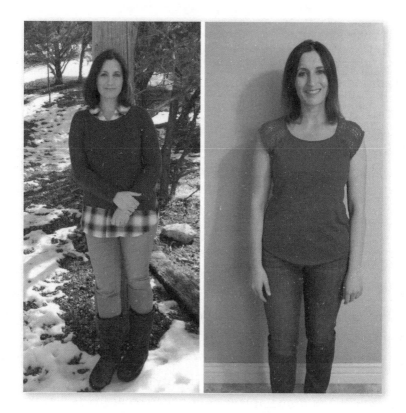

In summary, the 3X lifestyle is a commitment you make to yourself and to your family that demonstrates your focus on health. While embarking on this new journey, especially for others in addition to yourself, this promise and declaration to plan your healthy lifestyle is the missing step in most weight-loss programs and a major reason why most diets fail.

THE 3X LIFESTYLE

The word "lifestyle" was incorporated into the name of my program because the type of change your body needs in order to see results are changes that should be implemented for your entire life, not just a period of time. As a reminder, the majority of weight-loss programs are not realistic and cannot be sustained over time. As a result, they precipitate rebound weight gain because they never show you how to handle the reason your body gained weight in the first place. And as soon as you're done with the diet, cleanse, or challenge and go back to your normal life, you gain all the weight right back.

This is why you need a healthy **lifestyle**, one that can be implemented into your everyday life so that it becomes a normal part of your daily routine. This plan should not only be something that will help you lose weight initially, but will get you all the way to your goal weight. It should also be a lifestyle that you can easily maintain, even after you've lost all your weight.

When it comes to losing weight, most women just try to wing it, and they rely upon two things to get themselves through: their initial enthusiasm for the new diet or new exercise program, and then when that wears off, they try to rely simply on willpower. But enthusiasm and willpower are not enough to get you the results that you are looking for.

In order for you to be effective and to get results with your weight-loss effort, you need to have a plan of attack on how you are going to win the war on weight. Because it *is* a war and up until now, it's been a series of losing battles. By committing to 3X, you can take control of the entire process and greatly increase your chances of success.

Believe it or not, being proactive is directly related to your ability to stay on a healthy eating plan. Beginning an effective, realistic weight-loss plan that works for you can take some time getting used to at first. But once it's implemented, it becomes a normal part of your everyday routine, and you will find that you actually save a lot of time and money in the long run by planning ahead. Not to mention that you get to reap the rewards and the tremendous benefits that come from living a healthy lifestyle and losing weight that goes along with it.

I want you to picture something for just a moment.

It's Monday morning and you just woke up. You step on the scale and you're down another pound. You can't believe you are still losing weight. The time seems to go by so fast and this is the first time you've gone this long without cheating. You never dreamed it would be this easy. The healthy lifestyle you are living is effortless. It has become a routine, a normal part of your everyday life, and you never have to think about it.

You've been experiencing positive benefits of losing weight and getting healthy, such as improved digestion, less bloating, less gas, and more regular bowel movements. Your skin is clearer. You have much better sleep, more energy throughout the day, and a better mood. You've got more enhanced mental focus and have even lost four dress sizes and can now fit into your skinny jeans.

Everyone you know is complimenting you, telling you how great you look, begging you to tell them your secret. Little do they know that your body is on complete fat-burning autopilot. While everyone else is starving themselves and spending every spare moment of their time doing cardio at the gym, you're going through life normally, you're not stressed, you eat food when you want, you're not hungry, you don't have to fight cravings, and every day you wake up to find you've lost more weight.

Can you imagine that just in a few short weeks from now, this will be your lifestyle? Is it too good to be true? Absolutely not! You're going to see for yourself that all this and more is possible and is waiting for you at the end of the next few weeks.

Take a look at what some of my clients have said about living the 3X Lifestyle:

"3X is the back-to-basics clean-eating lifestyle."

"Feels clean inside and out, and puts me back in control of my body."

"The best, most healthful way to eat for fitness, weight loss, and health."

"Best and easiest plan to follow to feed your body to look and feel good inside and out."

"3X is a very simple, effective, and amazing lifestyle eating plan."

"Amazingly energetic and full of happiness for my future with my 3X Lifestyle."

"Don't be lied to. Being healthy is not complicated."

"With 3X, you never have to diet again. You eat when you want, and you make sane choices."

Join my clients and me in this 3X Lifestyle and live your best life!

CHAPTER 10

IT'S ALL ABOUT PREP

As we established earlier on, preparation is one of the keys to success with the 3X Program. So now is the point where you will make space in your life for the wholesome nutritious food that you will be consuming with your new healthy eating plan. This means getting rid of bad foods that you might currently have taking up space in your life. This step is **not** optional. It is a proven element to achieving success and can actually be very therapeutic.

First, go through your pantry and throw out anything that has expired, including seasonings. Seasonings, believe it or not, are only good for 6-12 months, even though most people (like my grandma) keep the same spices in their cabinet for their entire lives. This ensures that you're not causing yourself any unnecessary harm or adverse effects by eating something that should no longer be consumed.

Next, remove anything that was mentioned in the chapter on fat-storing foods from your pantry. This includes all processed foods like canned soups, snacks, and bottled condiments because these contain many ingredients that are harmful to your health and slow weight-loss results tremendously. Also remove vegetable oils, sugar, artificial sweeteners, and anything containing milk, wheat, soy, or corn.

Once you've done the pantry, go through your fridge and do the same thing. Throw out old food, wilted vegetables, expired food and condiments, and get rid of processed foods, dairy products, bread, and anything else on the fat-storing foods list. Once you've done this, consider donating these goods rather than throwing them away.

Then I want you to do something that will give you an extra clean start to the program, and that is clean your fridge. Pull out the drawers and wash them out with warm water, soap, and white vinegar. Wipe down all the shelves and the inside of the doors.

Now that your fridge is sparkling clean and your pantry is clear of all expired items and processed foods, it's time to plan your meals, go grocery shopping and re-stock your kitchen with freshly prepared food and healthy condiments and seasonings.

To restock your fridge, select your vegetables and protein by making sure that they are all organic, grass-fed, wild, or free-range. You want your food to be in as close to its original state as possible and minimally processed. No pesticides, hormones, antibiotics, nor processed meats.

Rewind the clock about 75 years and pretend you're a farmer and everything that you put onto your table came fresh from your farm. The ground soil where you planted your vegetable seeds were rich in nutrients and they were watered from the purest water source. The animals that were raised were treated with care and fed grass, not genetically altered soy and corn that have been doused with chemicals. You caught the freshest fish from the purest rivers, lakes, and oceans.

That is how we should be eating today as well if we want the best health possible! So try to seek out top quality food that has been raised with care. And remember, it's okay to invest in yourself! You deserve the best, so why not give the best for your body?

MEAL PREP MADE EASY

"By failing to prepare, you are preparing to fail."
-Benjamin Franklin

The term "meal prepping" is used to refer to the practice of planning and preparing your meals ahead of time. It is a proactive (meaning to prepare for in advance) approach to healthy eating. In this chapter, we are going to talk about how meal prepping can ensure your success on this program. I will explain exactly how to plan and prepare your meals so that you can save time, money, and your sanity, and then I will give you some helpful tips, suggestions, and meal-planning recipes to make your food-prep journey simple and easy.

Why take the time to meal prep? There are three main reasons:

1. When you take the time to plan and prepare, healthy food choices will become a no-brainer and facilitate you reaching your weight-loss goals.

2. Meal prepping eliminates the stress and frustration that can go along with adjusting to new habits and transitioning toward a healthy lifestyle, and it can determine the success of your weight-loss efforts.

3. Being organized through planning and preparing in advance will reduce your chances of failure due to not having anything to eat and deciding to go from non-optimal food choices.

The most important part of meal prepping is to keep it simple! When first starting out on a new eating plan, it is best to keep everything as simple as possible so that you don't unnecessarily overwhelm yourself. In order to do this, don't try a new recipe for every meal every day! Just because we are going to keep it simple doesn't mean it's not going to be fun and delicious though. We are starting out with baby steps. No need to worry about getting "bored" with your food.

You'll need to fully grasp how to prepare your food in advance so that you have a fully stocked kitchen at all times. We do this by starting with the basics and building from there. My advice is to be simple during the week and spice it up on the weekends with various recipes when you have more time and flexibility.

For the first few weeks, I suggest eating the same breakfast and lunch every day and then making three main dinner meals with enough leftovers for the alternate night's dinners. This way you do not have to cook a new meal every day.

Here is an overview of a simple, basic meal prepping strategy. Starting with meats, choose a variety of 3 for the week. Let's say you choose chicken thighs, salmon, and ground beef. I suggest cooking them all at the same time in the oven. It's fast and convenient and doesn't require washing a ton of dishes. Use different cooking sheets/trays and season each meat differently to change it up. You can also make double batches of each meat and freeze whatever you aren't going to use for the next 3 days.

In addition to cooking the protein, you can begin chopping vegetables for salads and cook vegetables for your dinners as well. Some examples are food processing cauliflower to make cauliflower rice, slicing carrots for carrot fries, or washing and slicing Brussels sprouts, asparagus, broccoli, etc. You can also spiralize zucchini for spaghetti. You can cook your prepped veggies ahead of time and reheat them when you're ready, or just wash and chop them so that they will be ready to cook upon mealtime. Organic frozen vegetables that can easily be steamed and seasoned are another option for an easy side dish.

You also will want to prepare your own condiments each week by making them yourself. Most bottled condiments from grocery stores are filled with bad oils, hidden sugars, and other chemicals and preservatives that can stop any weight loss. I suggest making your own salad dressings, sauces, and dips, using fresh or organic dried spices. Making these in advance so that you have them on hand is an easy way to make your food taste delicious without spending a lot of time in the kitchen cooking a gourmet meal.

Once you have your protein, vegetable, and healthy fat you can mix and match them into different meals and place them into glass containers so that when you are ready to eat, all you have to do is pull them out of the fridge. After you have three days' worth of meals you can freeze the rest and pull it out the day before you need it.

THREE STEPS TO SUCCESSFUL MEAL PLANNING

Step 1: Prepare your week

1. Set aside time to plan out the meals for the coming week.

2. Pull out your calendar for the next week and make your meal plan based on what you have scheduled. For example, if you have a lunch meeting on Tuesday at a restaurant with a new client, you know that you will not need to pack lunch for that day.

3. After you have your calendar ready, take a blank meal-planning calendar, get out your favorite recipes, and start filling in the calendar with what you plan to eat.

4. Once your meals are planned out for the week and you know what you will be having each day for breakfast, lunch, and dinner, it's time to create your grocery list based on the amount of food that you will need.

Step 2: Shopping

I like to spend the least amount of time going back and forth from the grocery store. This wastes a lot of valuable time and it is so much better to get everything all in one trip. Therefore, I recommend buying all the meat and frozen vegetables for the entire month in one trip and freezing everything. Then you only need to make a quick stop by the produce stand or grocery store once a week or even bi-weekly for your fresh vegetables for salads. This will eliminate the time spent at the grocery store and will always ensure you have enough food on hand.

Here are tips for maximizing your grocery shopping:

1. Make a base list of the basics. Things like chicken, beef, shrimp, fish, frozen vegetables, spices, condiments, etc. These are the common items that you will need to stock in your freezer and pantry so that you always have the basics on hand.

2. Add any additional specialty vegetables, seasonings, or ingredients that you will need for the week of recipes that you have planned to eat. Special herbs, vinegars, or oils that you may not necessarily have on hand as common items. These items, along with the weekly fresh vegetables, should be the only items you need to get on a weekly or bi-weekly basis.

3. Once you have gone shopping for the monthly base items (frozen meats, frozen vegetables, condiments, and seasonings) and have purchased your weekly (or bi-weekly) items, such as the fresh vegetables, herbs, and unique ingredients, it's time to prepare the food for the upcoming week!

4. I do not recommend shopping and prepping all in the same day because you might feel overwhelmed. I shop on

Saturdays and then prep my food on Sundays. It is up to you. If you shop and prep on the same day, make sure you have set aside the entire day because it will take a quite a bit of time to do both in the same day. Also, do not plan to shop and prepare your meals on the same day that you have an event to go to, or else you will end up seriously stressed.

Step 3: Prepare

This is the exciting part. As long as you have set aside the time to do nothing else but prep your entire kitchen, this is a very fun experience! I highly suggest allowing an entire day, or at minimum a half day for prepping. This way you do not get stressed about time.

Again, I highly recommend keeping it simple. Start by eating the same thing for breakfast and lunch every day. Then you can rotate three recipes for dinner during the week. For example, make a double batch of three main dinner meals for the week on Sunday. This will give you a total of six meals, which will last you Sunday through Friday. Eat Sunday's dinner that night, store Monday's and Tuesday's in the fridge, and freeze Wednesday's, Thursday's, and Friday's dinners. Be sure to take out the frozen meals the night before so they have time to defrost. You can even take this a step further and increase your batch to have enough for the following week's dinners, in which case you will have made enough meals for two weeks in one day! I highly suggest this method of prepping.

Another option, instead of cooking all the food for one to two weeks in one day (which could be an all-day affair), is to make a double batch of food every time you cook a meal during the week. For example, on Monday you decide to make turkey chili. You make a double batch and eat the first batch for dinner and store or freeze the second batch. Voila! Later on in the week, you already have another dinner prepared.

I absolutely could not live without my crock-pot! They are simple, do not require much preparation, and are my favorite types of meals to make. You can usually just take the meat and vegetables out of the refrigerator in the morning, throw them in the crock-pot with the spices, herbs, and sauces, set the crock-pot, and go about your day. When you come home in the evening, a nutritious, rewarding meal will be waiting for you. There are always plenty of leftovers also. Some sample crock-pot dinners include a roast with root vegetables, a whole chicken with vegetables, or turkey or beef chili.

That sums up my meal prepping system and strategies. I hope you find this valuable, and that you do not underestimate the power of being prepared.

CHAPTER 11

OVERCOMING CRAVINGS

The number one thing women struggle with when trying to eat healthy and lose weight is cravings. No surprise, right? Well, the amazing thing about 3X Weight Loss is that if you do it correctly and follow The Perfect Day, the cravings will completely go away. However, in order to experience this state of "no cravings," you have to fully eliminate all sugars because if there is any in the diet your body will burn sugar instead of fat and when it is in a sugar-burning state, you will continue to crave it. When you no longer crave sugar, it is an indicator that you are burning fat.

In this chapter, I am going to show you the different types of cravings that you need to be aware of so that you can easily do the program and switch your body from sugar-burning mode to fat-burning mode.

HABIT CRAVING

The first type of craving is called a "habit," which is a craving that occurs because of having established certain habits and eating patterns. Studies have proven that eating specific things stimulates a chemical in the brain that causes a desire for those same foods. Here's how it works: If you eat a piece of chocolate every night after

185

dinner, your brain will actually rewire itself and create a habit of this. Inevitably, you will crave chocolate every night after dinner.

The brain chemical responsible for this is called Neuropeptide Y (NPY). NPY causes the creation of new fat cells and fat to build up in the belly, causing weight gain. What's interesting is that the levels of NPY in your brain are triggered by your diet. You do *not* want high levels of NPY. The more NPY a person has, the more likely the person is to consume carbohydrate-rich food. And carbohydrates and sugar boost the production of this neurochemical NPY. So, the more carbohydrates and sugar you consume, the more NPY you have, the more you will crave these types foods, the more your body will make fat and the harder it will be to lose weight.

The flip side to that is that when you stop eating carbs and sweets, you will lower your NPY and stop craving these types of foods. That is what the 3X Program helps you do. It helps you establish those good habits so that you're no longer fighting the food addictions, cravings, bad junk food, and all the stuff that gets in the way of losing weight and being healthy.

There are a lot of other programs out there that tell you that you can still eat fat-free ice cream and wheat bread as long as you don't go over a certain number of calories. But when you do that, the ice cream or bread is causing you to have more and more cravings. This means you never break those bad food addictions and you will have to diet for the rest of your life because with those types of programs, you're not getting rid of any addictions.

All you're doing is tricking your body into losing weight in the short term by restricting calories, but you haven't actually broken the addictions to the very foods that caused weight gain in the first place.

ADDICTION CRAVING

The second type of craving is an addiction craving, which is very similar to the habit type of craving. This is the type of craving you get when you're eating processed foods that have a ton of MSG, chemicals, sugar, flavor enhancers, coloring, and artificial flavorings because all these things have very addictive properties. The food manufacturers put this stuff in the food so that we become addicted to it. So you have essentially hardwired your brain to want these types of foods and you are also becoming addicted to the sugar and chemicals that have been added to processed foods.

DEFICIENCY CRAVING

The third type of craving is deficiency cravings. Believe it or not, when you are deficient in certain nutrients like minerals and vitamins, you will start to have cravings because your body thinks it is starving. And nutritionally, it is! So what is it going to do? It's going to tell you, "Go eat! I'm starving." But it's not going to differentiate between a piece of broccoli and a piece of pizza. It's just going to say, "Eat!" If you also have habit cravings and addiction cravings when your body tells you to eat, then you're going to reach for the pizza, chocolate, or whatever you're addicted or used to eating. You're not going to reach for the broccoli or the spinach salad, which is what your body is really craving. When your body is nourished and satiated, cravings rarely exist. This is another reason why it is important to make sure you follow the food plan and The Perfect Day. It was designed intentionally to nourish your body and eliminate cravings that occur from nutrient deficiencies. You might still have the food addictions to break and habit cravings to overcome, but deficiency cravings will not be present if you follow the plan.

OVERCOMING THE 3 TYPES OF CRAVINGS

You need to know about these three types of cravings so that you can prepare for and handle them accordingly. We will address the habit cravings first, by breaking bad habits and creating new, healthy habits. On the 3X Weight Loss Program, you'll have a list of all of the healthy fat-burning foods and alternatives to bad foods that you can swap out so you can establish those new healthy habits.

I want you to start becoming aware of what's happening when you start to have a craving and recognize what it is. For example, when you have a huge craving for chocolate, you can spot what's happening and think, "Okay, it's that time of night when I always used to have a piece of chocolate. That's what's happening right now. My brain thinks I need to have this and it's really hard to fight that off."

The key to breaking a habit craving is to not give in, because every time you do you're solidifying that habit even more. But every time you don't give in, you're breaking the habit bit by bit.

A great way to break a bad habit is to replace it with a new, healthy habit. So if you are used to having ice cream after dinner, have something from the fat-burning foods list. The only way to get rid of addiction cravings is to stop eating those foods. That is why we remove certain foods at the beginning of the program: to break those addictions. And luckily, you'll find that pretty soon you won't even want those types of food because your body will start to crave healthy food.

Lastly, for the deficiency cravings, you need to give your body as many nutrients as you can so that it feels nourished. When it is nourished, it will not crave bad food as much. We do this with the fat-burning foods, the green juice, and the supplements.

Now that you understand the types of cravings, there are two very crucial things you must know about them. The first is that during the first few weeks, it is very important that you do not give into your body's cravings because if you do, you will be feeding a monster that will only get stronger and stronger every time you feed it. In other words, the cravings will not go away if you continue to hardwire your body into wanting bad foods.

The second thing to know is that if you cheat and eat any sugar, your body will not burn fat for three days (I keep reiterating that point because it is VERY important). When your body gets sugar, it immediately shuts off fat burning and goes into fat-storage mode, and takes roughly three days to get rid of all the sugar and get back into fat-burning mode. So if you cheat a couple of times a week, you will see that you will not be losing any weight.

It usually only takes 30 days to break through the cravings once and for all. This only happens if you do it right though. So my advice to you is to follow the 3X Program perfectly for 30 days straight, and you will not only lose weight quickly, but you will be forever free of the bad food habits and cravings that have kept you spinning your wheels in the diet trap for so long.

If it is very hard for you to tough it out and stick to the program without giving in to the cravings, I recommend the herbs and homeopathic remedies I talked about in the supplements section. In addition to taking these supplements, there are some other things you can do to help with cravings which I will mention below. They aren't going to eliminate the source of those cravings, which are habits, addictions, and deficiencies, but they will help you get through the program.

HANDLING CRAVINGS

The first thing that helps is to make sure you are getting enough healthy fats. This is a hard one at first because most women still believe that fat will make them fat. So instead of getting enough healthy fats, they leave them out and then end up feeling hungry or having more cravings. So my first piece of advice is to make sure you are getting your healthy fats. If you have a craving for something sweet, eat a tablespoon of coconut oil and I guarantee it eliminates the craving instantly. Coconut oil is also amazing for cravings because your body immediately uses it as fuel and it zaps cravings and hunger immediately.

One more trick to getting rid of cravings is taking a tablespoon of pine nut oil. Pine nut oil is one of the strongest *natural* appetite suppressants on the planet. Pine nuts and pine nut oil have a long history of suppressing appetite and boosting energy. Its use dates back to Greek and Roman times. Siberians, during the long winters where food was often scarce, have used pine nuts or a tablespoon of pine nut oil either with a meal or in some cases to replace a meal, as it contains pinolenic acid, which is known to produce a long-lasting feeling of fullness.

Pine nut oil has also been shown to help with lowering cholesterol and blood sugar levels, high-blood pressure and boosts immunity. It can also make you feel more energetic and it very effectively promotes weight loss.

Last but not least, I recommend a product called CALM, which you can buy at some grocery and health-food stores. It's a magnesium drink that you mix with warm water and drink like a tea, and it's good to drink before bed at night. It's sweetened with stevia, so there's no sugar in it, but it does have a very sweet flavor and kind of calms you down when you're feeling like you have to have some sugar.

Cravings really are the biggest struggle that we have when trying to lose weight and be healthy. But I promise you that if you follow these tips you are going to have a great experience on this program. And this is what I want for you, because I want to see you reach your weight-loss goal.

As a bonus, I have included some of my favorite healthy alternatives to sweets in the back of the book so make sure you check those out!

You are now in the home stretch! Continue on with me as I give you the tools to help you understand and conquer plateaus.

CHAPTER 12

BREAKING THROUGH A WEIGHT-LOSS PLATEAU

Sometimes people lose weight so fast at the beginning of their 3X journey that they think there is something wrong if later on in the month they go a week or two without seeing any changes on the scale. I am going to explain what is happening on the first few days on the program and why you will experience such rapid results in the first two weeks but then experience tapering results.

Anytime you have weight to lose, that weight is made up of water, toxins, and fat. For the first couple weeks on the program, you are losing a combination of water and fat, along with toxins and waste residue clogged in your intestines. As a result, the weight loss is more rapid at the beginning of the program. Once all the water weight is gone, you will see the number of pounds lost on the scale starting to slow down. Speaking of the scale, I actually recommend not weighing yourself daily and not only using the scale as a measure of success, because the fluctuations of the scale in the first few weeks will drive you nuts.

Now please note that this does not mean you aren't still burning fat. Also, if you lose a lot of weight in the first week, and then the second week you gain .5 pounds, it doesn't mean you gained .5 pounds of fat. It is just the water weight is only fluctuating, which is normal.

Another thing to recognize is that your body will burn fat in a direct ratio to your health, so some of you may lose weight faster, and some may have more healing to do before your body will lose a lot of weight. Please do not feel discouraged if you don't lose as fast as others; remember that everybody is different, and everyone heals at a different pace. Who knows? Maybe you are slower at losing weight in the beginning, but then later it picks up. Do not compare yourself to other people on the program. And do not quit because the answer to slow weight loss is *not to give up* and go off the program.

If any program is going to help you, it's going to be this one. So if you really want to handle your body issues and not continue to gain more and more weight and get unhealthier each year, then you need to be patient and stick to the program and not give up. This method will balance your hormones, reset your metabolism and heal your gut as long as you give it time to do so. Just keep doing it and you will see the results as your body starts to heal and when it feels safe, it will release the fat.

Following this program precisely and sticking to it without cheating eliminates real weight-loss plateaus. I define a weight-loss plateau as no change in how you feel, pounds lost, body fat percent or inches lost while being on the program for 30 days straight. A weight loss plateau is not being on the program for seven days without losing any weight or only losing one pound this week when you lost five pounds the week before. Even if you go a period of time without losing pounds on the scale, you will still be burning fat, losing inches, healing your body, and repairing your hormones and metabolism. Your body will always be working (and not just on losing weight), so be patient with it.

If, however, you honestly feel you have reached a plateau and you have been following the 3X Program to a tee (with no cheating) and are still having a hard time losing weight, here are some adjustments to make that can help:

1. Cut out all fruit, including berries.
2. Eat only three meals per day without snacking in between meals. If you find that you cannot make it to the next meal without feeling hungry, then you need more healthy fats with each meal.
3. Stop over-exercising (other than walking, yoga, swimming or biking for 20-30 minutes a day).
4. Start exercising if you haven't been (walking, yoga, swimming or biking for 20-30 minutes a day).
5. Cut out chicken. Focus on eating grass-fed beef and seafood only. This is because all chicken is fed soy, even if it is organic. Soy disrupts the hormones including the thyroid, which slows your metabolism.
6. Make sure you are getting enough to eat (at least 1,250 calories) every day.
7. Ensure you are drinking three to four liters of water a day (roughly a gallon).
8. Ensure you are getting eight hours of sleep each night. Fat burning takes place at night when you sleep, and will not happen if you are not getting enough quality sleep.
9. Make sure you finish eating three to four hours before going to bed and do not have a bedtime snack. Fat burning takes place during sleep and if your body is digesting food throughout the night, it won't burn fat, and you also will not be achieving good-quality sleep.
10. Are you drinking the green juice in the morning? If not, drink it.

11. Get 15-20 minutes of sunshine per day, your daily dose of vitamin D.

12. If you aren't taking omega-3 fish oil, you need to. This is to help lower inflammation in your body. Fat loss will be really hard in the presence of inflammation. If you have excess body fat, it is a sign of inflammation and you need to lower it.

13. Take all the supplements listed in the chapter on supplements. If you have had a hard time finding all the supplements that make this program the most effective, you can see the ones I recommend at www.3XWeightLoss.com/supplements.

14. If you have excessive cravings or hunger despite doing all of the above, you need more healthy fats. Follow the recommendations in the cravings section of this book.

15. Reduce your level of stress. Stress releases cortisol and cortisol stores fat. Cortisol also will convert your muscle into sugar, which will keep you from losing weight.

16. If you try all of the above and still can't lose weight, see a naturopathic doctor and have your hormones tested (even if you've had them tested before and they came back "fine"). Continue the 3X plan because eventually the program will correct imbalances, but you may need additional support (Chinese herbs, bioidentical hormones, etc.) that only a naturopathic doctor can prescribe with adequate testing.

17. You can also start your free trial of the 3X Weight Loss coaching program at www.3XWeightLoss.com/free-trial, which includes an additional course of study that is filled with knowledge to help you understand exactly what you need to do to make it through this journey and out the other side.

A FEW OF MY FAVORITE RECIPES

3X CHOCOLATE BROWNIES

Ingredients
- ½ cup ghee
- ½ cup coconut oil
- ½ cup of cocoa powder (unsweetened)
- 1 cup chopped walnuts
- ¾ cup xylitol or erythritol
- 4 eggs
- 1 tsp vanilla extract

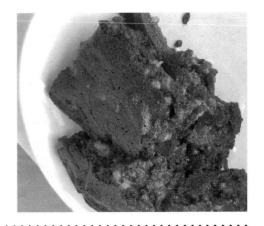

Directions:
1. Preheat oven to 375 degrees F.
2. Melt ghee and coconut oil.
3. On low speed, mix all ingredients until batter is smooth.
4. Grease an 8x8 square pan with coconut oil.
5. Pour mixture evenly into the baking pan.
6. Bake for 20 - 25 minutes or until done. Check brownies with a fork in the middle.
7. If the fork comes out clean they are done.
8. Let stand and cool for 15 minutes.
9. Keep remaining brownies in the fridge.

3X APPROVED SEED BREAD

Ingredients:
- 2 cups almond flour
- 7 eggs
- ½ tsp xanthan gum,
- ½ tsp sea salt,
- 1 tsp baking powder
- 1/4 cup of sunflower seeds
- 2 Tbsp. chia seeds
- 2 Tbsp. if coconut oil
- ½ cup of ghee
- 2 Tbsp. of sesame seeds to sprinkle on top

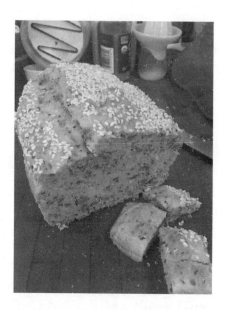

Directions:
1. Preheat oven to 350 degrees F.
2. Beat eggs and then mix in the half a teaspoon xanthan gum. Melt the ghee and coconut oil together and beat into eggs.
3. In another bowl, mix almond flour and the rest of the seeds and dry ingredients except the sesame seeds, which go on top at the end.
4. Mix the egg batter with the dry ingredients and stir until mixed well. Let sit for a few minutes until it thickens up.
5. Line an 8- or 9-inch loaf pan with wet parchment paper (because it's easier to mold) and put the dough in the pan. Sprinkle with sesame seeds and bake for 40 minutes or until the skewer comes out clean!
6. This toasts up great and is terrific with some avocado mash and cherry tomatoes with sea salt on top! It's almost all protein and fat! No carbs or sugar!

3X PANCAKES

Ingredients:

- 1 cup almond flour
- 1 Tbsp. xylitol
- ½ tsp baking powder
- ¼ tsp baking soda
- ⅛ tsp fine sea salt
- 1 egg
- 1 Tbsp. avocado oil (can also use walnut or olive oil)
- ½ cup coconut milk

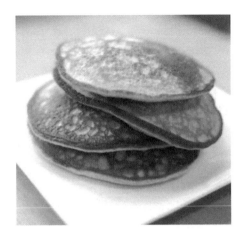

Directions:

1. Preheat griddle or pan.
2. Combine all dry ingredients and mix well.
3. Whisk egg and add avocado oil.
4. Add the coconut milk and stir.
5. Add the egg mixture to the dry ingredients and stir until smooth.
6. Allow batter to sit for a few minutes to rise.
7. Pour 4-8 small pancakes onto the griddle or pan.
8. Cook until edges are done, and bottoms are golden.
9. Serve hot.

3X ALMOND BUTTER FUDGE CUPS

Ingredients:
- ½ cup almond butter
- ½ cup melted coconut oil
- ¼ cup cocoa powder (unsweetened)
- ⅛ cup xylitol or erythritol sweetener

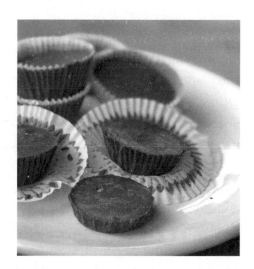

Directions:
Mix all ingredients together until smooth. Pour into little cups and put into fridge until hardens.

**For more recipes please visit
www.3xweightloss.com/recipes**

CONCLUSION

Congratulations! You've completed the book and are probably feeling excited, hopeful, informed, and...overwhelmed. Not only is that OK, it is expected. We covered a lot here, most of which was likely new information. You've just completed a full-on immersion in Weight Loss 101, and you should feel proud of yourself. You are now equipped with more knowledge and actionable information than 99.9% of the population and you know more now than most "experts."

As you embark on this 3X journey, keep this book nearby and refer to it often. It is your handbook. Again, you learned a lot here and it will take time before it is ingrained into memory. Having it handy will equip you to succeed when you're thinking about what foods to buy at the grocery store, which supplements are needed, etc. and make you less likely to slip up or cheat.

Making change is hardly ever easy, especially when it involves a lifestyle overhaul. So if you get discouraged, overwhelmed, or anxious, think about the reasons you sought out this book in the first place. If you made it to this point, you're telling me that you are serious about finally learning to properly care for your body and reaping the benefit of weight loss as a result. Remember that, be confident, know that every promise I made has been proven by my clients many times over, and that you can do it too!

And if along the way you feel like you need more support, you can start your free trial of the program where you can connect with other women on the program as well as get all the additional resources that are available to you as a 3X Weight Loss member.

Please visit http://www.3XWeightLoss.com/free-trial.

So what are you waiting for?! You now have all the information you'll need to change your life, packaged in the simplest way possible. Follow this plan, and your success is pretty much guaranteed! Go forth and conquer! I'm rooting for you and can't wait to share in your joy when you reach a milestone you never thought possible.

Your Weight Loss Coach,

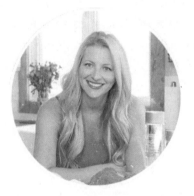

Laura Sales
Founder of 3X Weight Loss